CLINICAL LABORATORY ANIMAL MEDICINE

Clinical Laboratory Animal Medicine

AN INTRODUCTION

DONALD D. HOLMES, D.V.M.

The Iowa State University Press
AMES, IOWA

dedicated to my wife, Mary

Donald D. Holmes, D.V.M., M.S., is director, Laboratory Animal Resources, and professor, College of Veterinary Medicine, Oklahoma State University, Stillwater.

♾ Printed on acid-free paper in the United States of America from camera-ready copy supplied by the author

First edition, 1984
Second printing, 1987
Third printing, 1988
Fourth printing, 1990
Fifth printing, 1994
Sixth printing, 1995
Seventh printing, 1996

Library of Congress Cataloging in Publication Data

Holmes, Donald D.
Clinical laboratory animal medicine.

Bibliography: p.
Includes index.
1. Laboratory animals—Diseases. 2. Veterinary medicine. I. Title.
SF996.5.H65 1984 636.089 84-15768
ISBN 0-8138-0328-4

CONTENTS

PREFACE

The use of animal models in biomedical research is based on the axiom that fundamentally there is only one medicine for humans and animals. This might be paraphrased to "fundamentally there is but one veterinary medicine, whether the species under consideration is a horse or a hippopotamus, a mouse or a moose." The principles taught in both the preclinical and clinical phases of the veterinary medical curriculum apply to all animal species. By gaining familiarity with the more significant unique biologic features of laboratory animal species that are at times kept as family pets, learning of the more commonly seen disease processes, and applying knowledge and skills acquired during professional training, a graduate veterinarian should be capable of providing health care to these animals with a reasonable degree of competence that will improve with experience.

This book briefly describes unique anatomic and physiologic characteristics, the more common diseases, and recommended treatments for the species covered. In a modern, well-managed laboratory animal research facility, most of the conditions described would be considered uncommon if not rare. In this setting latent or subclinical viral infections, given scant attention in this book, are likely to be of greater concern than clinical disease, particularly in rodents. On the other hand, many of the bacterial, parasitic, and nutritional disorders described are not uncommonly encountered in pet animals or in animal colonies raised commercially for the pet trade or, in the case of rabbits, for meat.

The book does not presume to present clinical medicine of laboratory animals in the depth required by a specialist in laboratory animal medicine; rather, it has been prepared as an introduction for those planning to pursue further training in laboratory animal medicine, as a text for veterinary medical students, and as a practical guide to veterinarians in private practice. Actually, typical clinical laboratory animal veterinarians will devote more time to the treatment of random source traditional companion animals (i.e., dogs and cats) than the species described in this text, with the possible exception of nonhuman primates; nevertheless, they should acquire the skills necessary to provide appropriate health care to all species for which they are responsible.

The inclusion of reptiles and ferrets in this book is admittedly arbitrary, since neither are used in great numbers for biomedical or veterinary medical research. Their inclusion is due to an understanding that little information concerning ferrets and reptiles is presented in the veterinary medical curriculum at many institutions and the fact that these animals may be seen as patients in either a private practice or research setting.

Personal experience has revealed a general lack of enthusiasm by veterinary medical students for the study of nonhuman primates, presumably because only those anticipating careers as specialists in exotic or laboratory animal medicine expect to see nonhuman primates as patients. Although this view is understandable, a degree of familiarity with the species that most directly link veterinary and human medicine should, in this author's opinion, be an essential part of a laboratory animal medicine course presented to students pursuing the D.V.M. (or V.M.D.) degree.

With the increasing concentration of the nation's population in large cities and the resultant problems with confinement of the more traditional companion animals, the popularity of small mammals, reptiles, and birds is expected to increase. To undertake medical care of a species with which one is unfamiliar is unethical if not dangerous to the clinician as well as the patient; however, competence in the care of these species can be acquired without great difficulty and the results can be personally satisfying and profitable.

A note of caution might be injected at this point. The veterinarian treating systemic illnesses in the species described here can expect a lower survival rate than would be anticipated when treating the more familiar domestic animal species, and clients should be prepared for this reality. In maintaining the health of rodents, lagomorphs, nonhuman primates, and reptiles, a sound program of preventive medicine is much more rewarding than the treatment of such animals.

Some information is more readily comprehended when presented in the form of photographs or drawings rather than in words. For this reason, a review of colored photographic slides in the American College of Laboratory Animal Medicine and Science Series (which are available at most colleges of veterinary medicine and at many national professional meetings) is highly recommended for those wishing to further enhance their knowledge of laboratory animal medicine.

The efforts of Karen Walsh, Carri McLauchlin, and Carolyn Holmes in preparation of the manuscript are gratefully acknowledged.

CLINICAL LABORATORY ANIMAL MEDICINE

CHAPTER 1

MICE

CHARACTERISTICS

The common laboratory mouse is a rodent derived from the house mouse. Its scientific name is *Mus musculus*. More mice are used in research than any other mammal.

Genetic Types

Three genetic categories of mice are used in biomedical research: random bred, inbred, and F-1 hybrid. Random bred or outbred mice are produced in a large colony where matings occur randomly among males and females from unrelated litters. Random breeding should not be haphazard but planned in such a manner as to minimize inbreeding. Inbred mice are the result of brother-sister or parent-offspring matings. Twenty or more generations of brother-sister or parent-offspring matings are necessary to establish an inbred strain. F-1 hybrids are the progeny of matings between two inbred strains and are usually heartier than either of the parental strains. Mice within an inbred strain and F-1 hybrids are essentially identical genetically, thus eliminating an important variable in experimental work.

Uses

Relative to other species of research animals, mice are inexpensive to purchase and maintain and are therefore widely used in research studies and testing of various compounds for which large numbers of animals are required to provide statistically valid data. Millions of mice are used annually to test drugs and chemicals for toxicity and carcinogenicity.

Among the other favorable attributes of mice for research purposes are their short life span and great genetic diversity. A short life span permits the study of several generations over a period of a few years. Mutant strains of inbred mice provide investigators an almost unbelievable variety of animal models with which to study biologic processes and diseases. One example is the athymic nude mouse which is used extensively in immunologic research.

BIOLOGY

Anatomic Features

Brown fat tissue occurs in several places in the mouse. The most prominent masses are found between the scapula and are called the hibernating glands. Apparently, brown fat can be metabolized to increase heat production in response to exposure to a cold environment (McPherson 1973).

Mammary tissue is widely distributed in mice, with the glands extending well up onto the sides and back.

As in other rodents, the incisors of mice grow continuously and are worn down by friction.

Neonatal males may be distinguished from females by a greater anogenital distance, the pale testes visible through the abdominal wall, and larger genital papillae.

Physiology

Normal physiologic data are listed in App. 2.

The usual life span of a mouse is 1 1/2-3 yr. There are major longevity differences among strains.

White blood cell counts are highly variable. Even such factors as site of collection and time of day can influence the number of leukocytes in peripheral blood. For this reason, white blood cell counts are of little value in disease diagnosis.

Reproduction

Mating can usually be detected by the presence of vaginal plugs, which are formed by mixtures of secretions from the vesicular and coagulating glands of the male. The plugs usually persist for 18-24 hr but may last up to 48 hr. The usual gestation period in mice is 19-21 days and the usual weaning age is 18-21 days. The normal estrus cycle of females is 4 days when housed with males. Single females housed away from males cycle at 5 to 6-day intervals. Large groups of females housed together tend to go into anestrus and do not cycle; if these females are housed with males, they begin to cycle and 40-50% will be in estrus on the third day after introduction of a male. This synchronization of estrus is called the Whitten effect (Williams 1976). If a mouse bred within the previous 4 days is exposed to a strange male, the existing pregnancy will often be aborted. This phenomenon is known as the Bruce effect (Williams 1976).

Behavior

Adult males housed together will frequently fight and inflict severe wounds. The region around the genitals is often attacked. These wounds may become secondarily infected with *Staphylococcus aureus*. Bite wounds over the body must be differentiated from self-mutilation that results from mange mite infestation.

Drug Toxicities

Streptomycin and procaine are often toxic to mice even at low dosages and should therefore be avoided (Russell et al. 1981). Chloroform may also be toxic, causing liver and kidney lesions (Simmons and Brick 1970). Certain strains are particularly sensitive to chloroform, and males are more sensitive than females in some strains.

Husbandry

Mice may be housed in plastic (e.g., polycarbonate) or metal (usually stainless steel) shoe box style cages or in suspended metal cages with grid floors. A contact bedding material such as wood shavings or chips or particles of coarsely ground corncob are usually placed in the bottom of shoe box cages. An indirect bedding of absorbent material is frequently placed in waste trays located below cages with grid floors.

Food is usually provided in the form of commercially milled, firm, dry blocks fed ad libitum. Fresh, properly stored commercial diets from reputable companies are nutritionally complete in most cases. The food blocks should be placed in hoppers, either formed in the cage lid or attached to an inside cage wall. The practice of placing food blocks directly on the cage floor is both unsanitary and wasteful.

Water should be available continuously, either through water bottles with sipper tubes or automatic watering systems unless otherwise dictated by an experimental protocol.

In housing mice for research purposes, rigid control of room temperature, relative humidity, and lighting are essential. A temperature range of 70-74°F and a relative humidity of 40-60% is generally comfortable for mice and personnel providing their care. A constant cycle of darkness and light should be maintained in mouse rooms. Typically, a cycle of 12 hours darkness and 12 hours light is provided and is controlled by means of automatic timers.

The required frequency of cage cleaning depends to some extent on the number and size of mice caged together and the amount of air movement in the room; however, two to three times weekly is usually adequate. A musty odor is often evident in a room containing mice even when good cleaning practices are followed.

A detailed description of breeding practices in mouse colonies is beyond the scope of this book. Either a monogamous or a polygamous mating system may be established, with the choice of systems dependent on a number of factors. Breeding and preweanling mice should be housed in solid-bottom cages rather than in cages with grid floors. For maximum productivity, breeding should be commenced soon after animals reach sexual maturity and continued throughout the breeding life of the female. Difficulty may be experienced in inducing females to resume breeding if the breeding cycle is interrupted.

Recommended husbandry practices for rats, gerbils, hamsters, guinea pigs, and rabbits are similar to those described for mice except as noted in subsequent chapters.

TECHNIQUES

Handling and Restraint

To transfer a mouse from cage to cage, it may be picked by the base of the tail with bare fingers. If preferred, rubber-tipped forceps can be used to grasp a mouse either at the base of the tail or by the loose skin at the back of the neck.

The usual technique employed for holding a mouse to make an injection is to place it on a surface (such as a cage lid) to which it will cling; then grasp the tail with the thumb and forefinger of the right hand and, as the mouse attempts to move forward, grasp the skin at the back of the neck with the thumb and forefinger of the left hand and carefully but quickly gather the loose skin between these fingers. If the skin is held properly, the mouse can be lifted with the left hand and the tail secured between the small finger and palm. The right hand is then free to make the injection. Left handed persons may choose to alter the procedure so that the mouse is held in the right hand leaving the left hand free to make the injection.

Anesthesia

Anesthetic agents used in mice and recommended dosages are listed in section A.4 of App. 1.

Because of greater convenience and the small muscle mass in mice, inhalant anesthetics are more popular for procedures of short duration than agents designed for intramuscular injection. Furthermore, inhalant anesthetics permit better control of the depth of anesthesia than is possible with injectables. Ether and methoxyflurane are the commonly used volatile anesthetics.

A simple anesthetic chamber can be made by placing a ball of cotton containing ether or methoxyflurane in the bottom of a glass beaker and forming a platform of hardware cloth or similar material over the cotton ball to avoid wetting the patient with the anesthetic. Anesthesia is then induced by placing the mouse in the beaker and covering with a lid. When limb movement ceases and respiration is relatively slow and steady, the mouse should be removed from the chamber. If surgery is prolonged, anesthesia can be maintained by use of a nose cone made of paper or a plastic syringe cover having a small ball of cotton saturated with anesthetic at one end.

Pentobarbital, administered intraperitoneally, is sometimes used for procedures of longer duration. The dosage required for surgical anesthesia is quite variable and is influenced by the age and weight of the animal. The usual duration of anesthesia following pentobarbital administration is 20-40 min. For intraperitoneal injections the standard pentobarbital preparation should be diluted 1:10 using either sterile distilled water or physiologic saline; 0.7-1 ml of the diluted solution per 100 g of body weight should be administered. Because of the minute amounts required for mice, dilution of all injectable anesthetics is recommended.

Euthanasia

Methods of euthanasia commonly employed include administration of an anesthetic overdose, exposure to carbon dioxide in a closed chamber, and cervical dislocation. To separate the cervical vertebrae, the mouse is placed on a flat surface and an object such as a pencil is placed horizontally across the neck; then the mouse is pulled back quickly and firmly by the tail.

Medical Treatment

Because mice are so small, the evaluation of clinical signs is difficult and in many cases histopathology and microbiology are required for a definitive diagnosis. A binocular loupe and an otoscope are helpful in physical examination. Often mice must be treated symptomatically, and a rather high mortality can be expected with generalized infections.

Medication is usually administered by mixing into the water or feed. For greater accuracy or for unpalatable liquids, ball-ended dosing needles are useful. A tendency to overdose mice and other small rodents with injectable antibiotics is due to overestimation of their weight. Small scales (such as postage scales or a triple beam balance) are useful for obtaining accurate weights (Burke 1979). Dilution of drugs permits increased accuracy of dosage. Accuracy is further improved by use of tuberculin or insulin syringes. An incubator is useful in treating small rodents, particularly following surgery, because of the difficulty in maintaining normal body temperature.

BACTERIAL DISEASES

Bacterial and Mycoplasmal Pneumonia

Primary bacterial pneumonia is uncommon in mice unless the animals are immunologically deficient or stressed; however, bacteria are often cultured from pneumonic lungs of mice with primary viral or mycoplasmal infections. *Pasteurella pneumotropica* causes localized lesions in a wide variety of organs other than the respiratory tract and may play a role in respiratory disease under certain circumstances (Lindsey et al. 1982). Concurrent infection with *P. pneumotropica* and Sendai virus may result in fatal pneumonia (Harkness and Wagner 1983). Other bacteria that have occasionally been associated with respiratory disease in mice include *Klebsiella pneumoniae*, *Corynebacterium kutscheri*, and *Bordetella bronchiseptica* (Harkness and Wagner 1983). Infection with *Mycoplasma pulmonis* with or without concurrent bacterial or viral agents causes pneumonia in mice; however, murine respiratory mycoplasmosis is a much more serious problem in rats than in mice.

Signs associated with pneumonia include chattering, labored respiration, weight loss, and conjunctivitis. Treatment with antibiotics is frequently not practical in a research colony; however, antimicrobials such as chloramphenicol (Rx: A.1.b), ampicillin (Rx: A.1.a), or oxytetracycline (Rx: A.1.f) may be effective when circumstances justify their use.

For drug dosages, refer to the lettered and numbered notation in parentheses following Rx, which indicate sections in App.1 where suggested dosages are listed.

Salmonella spp. Infections

Salmonellosis was extremely common in mouse colonies at one time, but it now has been eliminated from most reputable breeding establishments by proper management practices. Colonies should nevertheless be continually monitored by periodic fecal culturing of live animals and by culturing, at necropsy, organs of animals dying of uncertain causes.

Salmonella infections may exist in mice as a latent or subclinical disease, and deaths occur as a result of flareups following stress (Williams 1976). Signs of acute or subacute disease include diarrhea, anorexia, weight loss, and a roughened hair coat. In animals dying of acute disease there may be an absence of gross lesions, or reddening of the distal ileum may be evident. Subacute to chronic disease is characterized by splenomegaly and the presence of yellow-white miliary foci in the liver, spleen, and lymph nodes (Ganaway 1982).

Antibiotic therapy does not produce bacteriologic cures; therefore, treatment is not recommended in case of an outbreak. Because of the danger of disease transmission by carrier animals and the zoonotic potential of *Salmonella* spp., affected colonies should be eliminated and equipment and rooms thoroughly decontaminated prior to introduction of clean stock.

Murine Colonic Hyperplasia

A variant of *Citrobacter freundii* may cause diarrhea and enterocolitis in mouse colonies. In natural outbreaks typical clinical signs include retarded growth, ruffled fur, soft feces, and occasional rectal prolapse (Ganaway 1982). The mortality rate is variable and depends on a number of predisposing factors.

The characteristic gross finding at necropsy is thickening of the distal half of the colon. Microscopically, mucosal hyperplasia, infiltration of inflammatory cells, and mucosal erosions may be evident in the affected portion of colon. Recommended treatments include neomycin (Rx: A.1.e), tetracycline (Rx: A.1.i), and sulfamethazine (Rx: A.1.h).

Pseudomonas sp. Infection

Mice that are irradiated or otherwise immunologically compromised are susceptible to a *Pseudomonas aeruginosa* septicemia and die an early death. "Early death" implies that death occurs prior to the anticipated radiation death time (i.e., 8 days or less). The course of *P. aeruginosa* septicemia is usually rapid, and clinical signs are limited to listlessness, anorexia, and death (Harkness and Ferguson 1982). In addition, otitis interna attributed to *P. aeruginosa* has been reported in mice in which no source of stress was evident (Kohn and MacKenzie 1980). These infections can be avoided by chlorinating the drinking water so that there are 10 ppm of free chlorine, using sodium hypochlorite (Rx: A.3.b) or acidifying to a pH of 2.5-2.58 with hydrochloric acid (Rx: A.3.a). Because of variations in water supply, acidity of the solution should be tested before use.

Tyzzer's Disease

Mice, as well as several other animal species, are susceptible to Tyzzer's disease caused by *Bacillus piliformis*. Tyzzer's disease usually occurs in animals housed under unfavorable conditions or immunosuppressed. Clinical signs may include diarrhea, dehydration, and anorexia; or animals may be found dead in the absence of obvious signs of illness. The disease occurs more frequently and is usually more severe in recently weaned animals (Harkness and Ferguson 1982). Gross lesions seen at necropsy include miliary, white to yellowish gray foci throughout the liver and at times a slightly reddened lower intestinal tract (Ganaway 1982). Treatment with antibiotics is frequently not effective; however, favorable results have been reported using tetracycline in the drinking water at high dosages (Rx: A.1.i) for 4-5 days.

Miscellaneous Bacterial Diseases

Streptococcus spp. infections are associated with dermatitis, pharyngitis, cervical lymphadenitis, bacteremia, and a variety of other disease processes. Systemic antibiotics and improved sanitation may be beneficial in treatment (Russell et al. 1981).

Staphylococcus aureus infections are most frequently associated with abscesses and skin lesions. Furunculosis caused by *S. aureus* is a particularly troublesome condition in genetically nude mice (McBride et al. 1981). Treatment is rarely successful.

Streptobacillus moniliformis infections are not common in mice but may occur in the form of either a generalized infection or an arthritis (Carlton and Hunt 1978). Penicillin (Rx: A.1.g) may be effective in treatment of these infections.

Corynebacterium kutscheri produces a disease termed pseudotuberculosis, which is characterized by the presence of disseminated abscesses (McClure et al. 1978). An acute form with high mortality may also occur (Harkness and Wagner 1977). Treatment is usually not successful.

VIRAL DISEASES

Ectromelia (Mousepox)

Ectromelia is very uncommon in the United States but is important when it does occur because it may be associated with high morbidity and mortality. The cost of an outbreak at the National Institutes of Health was estimated at $1 million (Held 1981b). The disease is usually introduced through importation of mice, tumor transplants, or other biologic material.

Mousepox infections may be latent, acute, subacute, or chronic. Clinical signs of the acute form include hunched posture, rough hair coat, conjunctivitis, facial swelling, and death. The subacute and chronic forms of ectromelia are characterized by a generalized body rash, swelling, necrosis and sloughing of appendages, and sporadic deaths (Harkness and Wagner 1977).

Diagnosis of the disease may be confirmed by the presence of intracytoplasmic eosinophilic inclusion bodies in the epithelial cells of the skin, small intestine, and pancreas. Serology and fluorescent antibody tests are also useful in diagnosis, particularly in latent infections.

There is no treatment for ectromelia. Vaccination may be feasible as a means of prevention in valuable colonies. Vaccine is administered by scarification of the tail, using human smallpox vaccine and a 26-gauge needle. Vaccine may be obtained from the National Cancer Institute (Wagner and Daynes 1981).

Sendai Virus

Sendai virus infection is the most common cause of viral respiratory disease in mice. It usually exists as an inapparent infection but may produce acute, sometimes fatal disease, particularly in suckling or weanling mice. There is a distinct strain variation in susceptibility to infection (Parker and Richter 1982). Sendai virus infection suppresses the normal antibacterial activity of the lungs, thereby predisposing infected mice to secondary bacterial pneumonia (Parker and Richter 1982). Clinical signs include a hunched posture, ruffled fur, dyspnea, and chattering. The severity of disease is intensified by secondary bacterial infection and immunosuppression. A killed vaccine of duck embryo origin is available commercially (Harkness and Wagner 1983). Antibiotics should be of benefit in preventing or eliminating secondary bacterial infection.

Infantile Diarrhea

Epizootic (or epidemic) diarrhea of infant mice (EDIM) and lethal intestinal virus of infant mice (LIVIM) are viral diarrheal diseases that occur in suckling mice. EDIM, the more common of the two, usually occurs at less than 2 wks of age and is characterized by the presence of soft yellow feces or an accumulation of dried feces around the anus. Affected mice usually continue to nurse (Kraft 1982). LIVIM may produce clinical signs up to 20 days of age. The mortality rate of LIVIM tends to be higher than EDIM, and the stomachs of affected animals are usually empty because nursing ceases with the onset of illness.

Spread of EDIM and LIVIM within a colony can be prevented by use of filter-top cages.

Lymphocytic Choriomeningitis

Lymphocytic choriomeningitis virus (LCM) is the only latent virus of mice that naturally infects man. Mice may serve as long-term asymptomatic carriers of the virus. Humans may acquire the infection by contact with tissue, feces, or urine of infected animals (Fox and Brayton 1982).

LCM infections in mice are usually asymptomatic, although both acute and chronic forms of the disease may exist. Signs of acute infection include decreased growth, rough hair coat, hunched posture, blepharitis, and convulsions (Harkness and Wagner 1983). An immune complex glomerulonephritis may develop with the chronic or persistent tolerant form of disease.

Miscellaneous Viral Infections

Mice are susceptible to a vast number of viral infections including K-virus, pneumonia virus of mice, reovirus type 3, mouse hepatitis virus, Theiler's encephalomyelitis, mouse adenovirus, and lactic dehydrogenase virus. These are primarily of concern as potential variables in biomedical research, and clinical signs are rarely seen in animals beyond the age of weaning.

PARASITIC DISEASES

Mites

Mites are very common in conventional mouse colonies. Although the degree of pathogenicity is highly variable, light infestations are usually inapparent, while heavy infestations cause dermatitis, alopecia, greasy-appearing hair, and self-inflicted trauma (Flynn 1975). An allergic component may be involved. Mite lesions must be differentiated from fight wounds, ringworm, and other skin disorders.

The more common species of pelage-inhabiting mites are *Myobia musculini*, *Radfordia affinis*, and *Mycoptes musculinus*. These mites may be detected by skin scrapings, but more conclusive results are achieved by killing the mouse and collecting mites as they leave the carcass. Various techniques are used to collect mites. One method is to remove the mouse skin and place it in a petri dish; after several hours discard the skin and examine the bottom of the dish under low magnification. Or the entire carcass can be placed in a high-walled glass jar, which is examined after the carcass has cooled. If mites are present, they can be transferred to a glass slide for identification.

Psorergates simplex is a follicle-inhabiting mite that produces dermal pouches appearing as small white nodules on the visceral surface of the skin. Lesions can be detected by removing the skin from a mouse and examining the inner surface for microscopic pouches (Flynn 1973).

Although treatment will reduce the mite population, complete eradication of mites without destroying an infected colony is unlikely. Among the treatments used with varying degrees of success are the following:

1. DDVP strips (Vapona) containing dichlorvos.
   a. Cut strips into 1 to 2-inch squares and place on top of cages for 24 hr at several weekly intervals (Harkness and Wagner 1977).
   b. Hang a DDVP strip from a rack of cages and cover the rack, cages, and strips with a painter's drop cloth for 24 hr. Generally, three treatments at 2-wk intervals are sufficient (Rush 1982).
2. Add 1/2 level teaspoon of Atgard V to bedding, fresh each week, for 2 wk (Williams 1976).
3. Apply dusts (e.g. 3-5% malathion) to animals and bedding or submerge in a dip (e.g. 0.5% methoxychlor).
4. Canex and mineral oil (1:4) applied to lesions with a cotton swab was found effective against *Radfordia affinis* (Stein 1981).
5. Cedar wood chips added to bedding are thought to be helpful in reducing the mite population (Williams 1976).

Pinworms

Pinworms (*Syphacia obvelata* and *Aspiculuris tetraptera*) inhabit the cecum and colon and are the most common nematode parasites that affect mice (Flynn 1973). *S. obvelata* is the more prevalent and troublesome. In most cases clinical signs are absent; however, heavy infections may lead to anal pruritis, rectal prolapse, and diarrhea. Neither are transmissible to humans.

The banana-shaped ova of *S. obvelata* can be detected by pressing a strip of cellophane tape to the perianal area, applying the tape to a glass slide, and examining under a microscope. The more oval eggs of *A. tetraptera* are detected by fecal examination.

Anthelmintics effective in treating pinworms include piperazine adipate (Rx: A.2.f), pyrivinium pamoate (Rx: A.2.g), dichlorvos (Rx: A.2.a), dithiazanine iodine (Rx: A.2.i) mebendazole (Rx: A.2.d) and Trichlorfon (Rx:

A.2.i). Complete elimination of *S. obvelata* without repopulation and strict sanitation is unlikely to be achieved.

Tapeworms

Hymenolepis nana, the dwarf tapeworm, is rather common in conventional mouse colonies. Mice may also harbor *H. diminuta*. Although both are potentially transmissible to humans, only *H. nana* is of practical public health concern since *H. diminuta* requires an intermediate host such as a grain beetle.

Diarrhea and retarded growth may occur with heavy infections, but most cases are clinically silent. Infections can be detected by the presence of ova upon fecal flotation. The recommended treatment is niclosamide (Rx: A.2.e). Eradication by means other than repopulation is extremely difficult (Flynn 1973).

Flagellates

Spironucleus (Hexamita) muris is a flagellate that occurs in the small intestine and cecum. In young animals the parasite may cause diarrhea and occasionally death, but it is less pathogenic in older animals (Flynn 1973). Treatment with dimetridazole (Rx: A.2.b) or oxytetracycline (Rx: A.1.f) is reported to be effective.

Rickettsia

Eperythrozoon coccoides is a rickettsial parasite of red blood cells. Normally, the parasite exists in a latent state; however, splenectomy of an infected mouse will precipitate a transient parasitemia and anemia.

MISCELLANEOUS CONDITIONS

Hair Loss

Mice frequently develop bilaterally symmetrical areas of alopecia on the muzzle caused by friction from bars on the feeder. Another cause of hair loss is barbering by cage mates. Most frequently, this hair chewing involves the vibrissae or the head region.

Water Deprivation

Water deprivation should not be overlooked as a possible cause of acute death in mice. Water may be unavailable because of an air lock in the sipper tube even when a water bottle is full. Malfunction of drinking valves in automatic watering systems can also result in a lack of water.

Neoplasia

The incidence and types of tumor occurring in mice are highly strain and age related.

CHAPTER 2

RATS

CHARACTERISTICS

Genetic Types

The laboratory rat most commonly used in research is derived from the Norway rat. Its scientific name is *Rattus norvegicus*. Rats may be either outbred or inbred. Outbred rats are usually spoken of as "stocks" and inbred varieties as "strains." Some of the common stocks or varieties of rats used in laboratories are the Sprague Dawley, Wistar, and Long Evans. Sprague Dawley and Wistar rats are albinos. The Long Evans is a hooded rat and is smaller and more aggressive than the other two varieties.

Ecological Types

In addition to the genetic types of rats, there are varying ecologic types (i.e., based on microbiologic status). These are germ-free or axenic, which are free of all detectable microflora; gnotobiotic, which have specified associated microflora (known flora); specific pathogen-free, which are free of specific pathogens (particularly *Mycoplasma pulmonis*); and conventional, or animals with undefined microflora (Baker 1977).

Uses

Although many people find rats distasteful, they actually make quiet, intelligent, easily trained, and gentle pets. They seldom bite unless provoked and do not have the distinct musty odor that is characteristic of mice.

Rats rank second only to mice in number used in biomedical research; rats and mice combined account for 14 times all other mammalian species used (Baker 1977).

BIOLOGY

Anatomic Features

Unique features of rats include the absence of a gallbladder, presence of a diffuse pancreas, lack of tonsils, and presence of numerous glands and glandlike organs in the head and neck (Baker and Bivin 1977).

As in other rodents, the incisors of rats grow throughout life and are continuously worn by abrasion of the occlusal surface. Malocclusion results in failure to wear off and consequent overgrowth of incisors (Baker and Bivin 1977).

Mammary tissue is very extensive, reaching between the forelegs, up to the shoulders, and back between the hind legs toward the vulva. With this distribution, mammary tumors may be found over a wide area of the body.

The cecum is highly developed and has a rumenlike function for microbial digestion of cellulose. In germ-free rats, the cecum may become greatly distended and occassionally twists on its long axis, resulting in fatal cecal torsion.

Males have a larger genital papilla and greater anogenital distance than females.

Physiology

Normal physiologic data is listed in App. 2.

The usual life span of a rat is 2-3 yr. Gnotobiotic and specific pathogen-free rats may live beyond 3 yr while conventional rats usually live no more than 2 yr because of spontaneous diseases. There are also considerable strain differences in longevity.

Reproduction

Rats reach puberty at 6-8 wk of age, but they are normally not bred until about 3 mo.

The usual gestation period of a rat is 20-22 days. If conception occurs during the postpartum estrus, the gestation period may be prolonged for 3-7 days because of delayed implantation (Harkness and Wagner 1977).

The usual weaning age of rats is 21 days.

Breeding animals are best housed in solid bottom cages containing wood shavings or other suitable bedding material. Either a monogamous or a polygamous breeding system may be followed. With a monogamous mating system, one male and one female are permanently paired and the offspring are removed when they reach weaning age. A polygamous mating system typically entails the housing of one male and two or more females together and removing pregnant females prior to parturition. Females are returned to the breeding cage after their litters are weaned.

HUSBANDRY

Nutrition

Rats grow, reproduce, and are maintained well on a standard commercial rodent diet, usually in the form of firm dry blocks or pellets, without any type of supplemental feeding.

Environmental Requirements

The temperature in the room used for housing rats should be maintained within a range of 70-74 °F and the humidity should be between 30 and 70%. Ventilation in a rat room should provide 10-15 complete air changes each hour with no recirculation of air unless it is properly filtered to remove contaminants.

Rats are nocturnal and must be provided with regular light/dark cycles for normal behavior and physiologic processes. In the laboratory, the light cycle is usually controlled by a timing device. Normally, 12-14 hr of light is provided daily. If regular light cycles are not maintained, the circadian rhythm will be disrupted, resulting in inconsistent responses to experimental manipulation (Baker and Bivin 1977).

Light intensity, noise, and various chemicals and drugs have a profound effect on experimental data. Pesticides are of particular concern because of their effect on hepatic microsomal enzyme activity. Cedar shavings used as bedding also affect hepatic microsomal enzymes. A method of estimating hepatic microsomal enzyme activity is to measure sleeping time following administration of pentobarbital. Biochemical tests are employed for more precise measurements of hepatic microenzyme activity.

Housing

Rats are ordinarily housed in metal cages with wire mesh bottoms or shoe box-type cages constructed of plastic or stainless steel. Shoe box cages may be covered with fiberglass filters to reduce infectious disease transmission and irritation from dust. The value of filter tops is offset to some extent by the fact that they permit high ammonia concentrations and increased temperature and humidity in the interior of the cage.

TECHNIQUES

Handling and Restraint

Rats are usually handled with bare hands. Heavy leather gloves that are too thick for the rat to bite through are awkward to use. A hand towel can be wrapped around the body of the rat to avoid the risk of being bitten while giving an injection.

Rats should not be carried or lifted by the tail because the skin may slip off; however, the tail may be grasped at its base as the initial step in picking up a rat. When the rat attempts to move away, the hand is placed firmly over the back and rib cage, restraining the head with the thumb and forefinger immediately behind the mandible.

Plastic cylinders and other devices can be used to restrain rats. These have openings to permit injections, blood collection, and other manipulations.

Blood Collection and Intravenous Injections

Small volumes of blood can be obtained by amputating or incising the tip of the tail. To facilitate the procedure, the tail is immersed in warm water or warmed with a light bulb for a few minutes to dilate the caudal vessels. Injections in young rats can also be made using the tail vein. Other methods for collecting small amounts of blood include penetrating the orbital sinus with a capillary tube or snipping a toenail. Larger volumes of blood may be obtained by cardiac puncture of an anesthetized rat.

Urine Collection

Urine can be collected by placing rats in specially designed metabolism cages. These enclosures have feed and water containers outside the cage and devices for separating urine and feces below.

Oral Medication

Drugs can be administered by incorporating the medication in the water or feed if the taste is not unpleasant. Sugar or syrup (1 tsp/L drinking water) will improve the palatability. A ball-ended dosing needle can be used for individual liquid medication.

Anesthesia

Agents commonly used for anesthesia and recommended dosages are listed in section B.4 of App. 1.

Of the inhalant anesthetic agents, methoxyflurane and halothane are preferable to ether. Ether is irritating to the respiratory tract, and this is particularly undesirable in rats with respiratory disease.

Systems for induction of anesthesia using volatile agents include use of

(1) a covered glass beaker with a cotton ball containing the anesthetic placed in the bottom (hardware cloth should be positioned over the cotton ball to prevent wetting the rat), (2) a face mask made from a disposable plastic syringe case containing a cotton ball saturated with the anesthetic (this technique is more useful for maintaining anesthesia than for induction), and (3) a plastic bag attached to the outflow hose of an anesthetic machine.

Euthanasia

An overdose of a barbiturate solution or ether is commonly used for euthanasia. A more convenient and economical method is the use of a carbon dioxide chamber, which can be constructed from an aquarium or other clear plastic enclosure. This system is also suitable for producing anesthesia of short duration.

At times animals must be killed without the possibility of complications resulting from anesthetics or euthanizing drugs. In such cases, rats can be killed by decapitation with a guillotine. Although lacking aesthetic qualities, the procedure is humane if properly performed.

BACTERIAL AND MYCOPLASMAL DISEASES

Chronic Murine Pneumonia

Synonyms for chronic murine pneumonia include chronic respiratory disease, murine pneumonitis, infectious catarrh, enzootic bronchiectasis, and murine respiratory mycoplasmosis. The latter term is becoming increasingly popular.

Mycoplasma pulmonis is the primary etiologic agent; however, other viruses and bacteria are often recovered from the lungs of infected animals. Rats are the most common host for *M. pulmonis* respiratory infection and this is by far the most common disease of laboratory rats. Mice are also susceptible to infection but much less so than rats. Rats are usually infected shortly after birth by exposure to infected dams. Such factors as high ammonia levels, other respiratory irritants, and various forms of stress have a profound effect on the clinical course and severity of the disease.

The disease is usually slowly progressive, with young animals only mildly affected but clinical signs becoming more severe in older animals. Clinical signs are typically not evident until an advanced stage of disease is reached. A serous or catarrhal nasal and ocular discharge may occur; but the sound of snuffling is usually more obvious than other early clinical signs. Animals with extensive pulmonary involvement may exhibit labored breathing, weight loss, lethargy, a hunched posture, and a rough hair coat. Acute deaths are usually the result of secondary bacterial infections.

Unilateral or bilateral otitis interna (labyrinthitis), characterized by the presence of a head tilt, is part of the chronic respiratory disease syndrome. It occurs because of an extension of the infection up the eustachian tube into the middle ear and then to the inner ear. When rats with labrinthitis are held by the tail in a vertical position, they typically rotate their bodies rapidly; whereas rats without inner ear involvement remain rigidly suspended (Cassell et al. 1979).

In the earliest stage, pulmonary lesions are limited to peribronchiolar lymphoid hyperplasia, visible only on microscopic examination of the lung. As the disease progresses, well demarcated foci of firm red-gray consolidation appear. Later, inflammatory debris and mucus accumulate in the air passages, resulting in bronchial distention and producing bulging yellow foci that in some cases give the lung a cobblestone appearance.

Diagnosis is based on history, clinical findings, gross and microscopic lesions, and isolation of *M. pulmonis* from the nasopharynx, tympanic bulla, trachea, or lungs (Harkness and Wagner 1977). In addition, an enzyme-linked immunosorbent assay test kit is now available for detection of *M. pulmonis* infection (Mia et al. 1981).

Antimicrobials added to the drinking water for periods of a week or more will suppress *M. pulmonis* infection but will not eliminate the disease. Bacterial culture and sensitivity testing are necessary to determine the most appropriate choice of antibiotics. Oxytetracycline (Rx: B.1.f) or tetracycline (Rx: B.1.i) in the drinking water are commonly used. For treatment of individual animals, chloramphenicol (Rx: B.1.b) or tylosin (Rx: B.1.j) may be injected intramuscularly for 5 days or more). Labyrinthitis does not usually respond to treatment, but animals with pronounced head tilt will often survive for months.

Elimination of this disease requires cesarean derivation of breeding stock and maintenance of animals under a barrier system.

Streptococcal Pneumonia

A common cause of bacterial pneumonia in rats is *S. pneumoniae*. Many rats harbor the organism from an early age, and disease outbreaks occur following stress such as transportation (Burke 1979). An increase in the incidence of acute respiratory disease in rats caused by *S. pneumoniae* has occurred in recent years (Weisbroth 1979).

Affected animals exhibit depression, a serosanguinous to mucopurulent nasal discharge, a snuffling respiratory sound, dyspnea, an ocular discharge, and ruffled fur. The disease tends to be acute to subacute and primarily affects younger animals (Weisbroth 1979).

Gross lesions often found at necropsy include seropurulent and fibrinopurulent pleuritis, pericarditis, epicarditis, peritonitis, meningitis, otitis media and interna, metritis, and bronchopneumonia (Harkness and Wagner 1983). A fibrinopurulent peritonitis and pleuritis with minimal involvement of the lung parenchyma is not uncommon.

Penicillin administered intramuscularly or in the drinking water (Rx: B.1.g) and oxytetracycline in the drinking water (Rx: B.1.f) are among the more frequently used antibiotics. Many others including ampicillin (Rx: B.1.a), chloramphenicol (Rx: B.1.b), and gentamicin (Rx: B.1.c), are also generally beneficial. The selection of an antibiotic is best based on the results of in vitro sensitivity testing. A carrier state often develops following treatment, and rats may experience a relapse during a subsequent period of stress.

Staphylococcal Infections

Staphylococcus aureus causes a variety of lesions in rats, including ulcerative dermatitis and poditis (Russell et al. 1981). Clipping of the toes or toenails is beneficial in eliminating the self-mutilation often associated with ulcerative dermatitis. Good sanitation procedures and in some cases antibiotics should be used along with toenail trimming to treat Staphylococcal infections.

Miscellaneous Bacterial Infections

Streptobacillus moniliformis is considered a commensal of low pathogenicity for rats (Weisbroth 1979) but is capable of producing disease in mice, guinea pigs, and humans. The organism is normally found in the nasopharynx of rats.

Pseudomonas aeruginosa is usually not pathogenic in immunologically competent animals, but the organism may become septicemic in animals following treatments that compromise the immune system (Weisbroth 1979). Chlorination of the drinking water (Rx: B.3.c) effectively protects animals against a *P. aeruginosa* septicemia.

Bacillus piliformis (Tyzzer's disease) occasionally occurs as an acute epizootic disease in rats (Weisbroth 1979).

Corynebacterium kutscheri, while usually existing as a latent or subclinical infection, may produce a subacute respiratory disease with abscesses in the lungs and less frequently other organs such as the liver and kidney (Weisbroth 1979). In chronic cases the abscess contents in the lungs become caseous, hence the term "pseudotuberculosis." The organism is sensitive to a wide variety of antibiotics, including ampicillin (Rx: B.1.a), chloramphenicol (Rx: B.1.b), and tetracycline (Rx: B.1.i); however, if the infection exists in an acute form, the rapid course may render treatment of individual animals ineffective (Harkness and Wagner 1983).

Salmonella spp. infections may exist in a latent subclinical form or cause acute disease with a high mortality. Clinical signs may include anorexia, rough hair coat, light soft feces, dyspnea, and an ocular discharge (Harkness and Wagner 1983). Congestion of the liver and spleen and thickening of the ileum and cecum are typical gross findings in animals dying of acute disease (Weisbroth 1979). Salmonella infections are uncommon in well-managed animal facilities, but with the possibility of introduction by wild rodents a program of periodically monitoring the colony for evidence of infection should be maintained. Treatment is usually not attempted because of the risk of survivors becoming carriers.

Pasteurella pneumotropica is gaining recognition as a significant pathogen of rats. Although usually existing as a latent infection, it may produce disease, acting either as a primary pathogen or a secondary opportunist with other agents such as Sendai virus or *Mycoplasma pulmonis* (Weisbroth 1979). Although clinical signs are usually those of pneumonia or an upper respiratory infection, abscesses of the skin, subcutaneous tissue, mammary glands, and other organs are occasionally caused by *P. pneumotropica* (Harkness and Wagner 1983). Chloramphenicol (Rx: B.1.b) may be beneficial in controlling clinical manifestations of infection (Weisbroth 1979).

VIRAL DISEASES

Sialodacryoadenitis

The coronavirus that causes sialodacryoadenitis is widespread in the rat population and may be found even in the colonies of reputable breeders. Clinical disease usually occurs either as an endemic infection of breeding colonies or as an explosive outbreak among nonimmune rats (Jacoby et al. 1979). The usual signs of infection are eye squinting, swelling of the ventral cervical region and jaw, and protrusion of the eye. Keratoconjunctivitis is the only clinical sign of infection in some outbreaks (Jacoby et al. 1979). Affected rats usually remain active and continue to eat (Harkness and Wagner 1983).

Although sialodacryoadenitis may spread rapidly in a susceptible colony, mortality is usually very low. Treatment is not indicated unless protrusion of the eyeball leads to keratitis, for which a topical ophthalmic preparation is indicated. Generally the swelling subsides in 10-14 days, and the rat returns to normal (Williams 1976).

Miscellaneous Viral infections

A number of viruses, including rat parvovirus, cytomegalovirus, rat coronavirus, and Sendai virus, produce natural infections in rats but are usually asymptomatic (Jacoby et al. 1979). Latent or indigenous viruses that may be activated by stress or alter the response of animals to experimental procedures are nevertheless of concern in the research laboratory.

PARASITIC DISEASES

Pinworms

Syphacia muris, *S. obvelata*, and *Aspiculuris tetraptera* are the pinworms of rats, with *S. muris* being the most common. None ordinarily cause clinical symptoms (Hsu 1979). The eggs of *S. muris* and *S. obvelata* can be detected in infected rats by microscopic examination of cellophane tape pressed against the perianal region. *A. tetraptera* infections are diagnosed by the presence of eggs in the feces or adult worms in the intestine (Hsu 1979). Sound management practices are required to prevent the introduction of pinworms into a colony. Piperazine (Rx: B.2.e; Rx: B.2.f), pyrivinium pamoate (Rx: B.2.g), and dichlorvos (Rx: B.2.a) are used in treatment, but pinworms are very difficult to eradicate.

Tapeworms

The rat is a definitive host for *Hymenolepis nana* and *H. diminuta*. These worms are pathogenic only with heavy infections; however, *H. nana* is of public health significance (Hsu 1979). Prevention of hymenolepid infections requires strict sanitation practices and elimination of vectors. Niclosamide (Rx: B.2.c) and quinacrine (Rx: B.2.i) are reported to be effective in treating rat tapeworms.

Urinary Bladder Worm

Trichosomoides crassicauda may be found in the urinary bladder or renal pelvis of rats (Hsu 1979). It is usually of no clinical significance (Williams 1976). Treatment with nitrofurantoin (Rx: B.2.d) or methyridine (Rx: B.2.b) is effective.

Flagellates

Spironucleus (Hexamita) muris is an enteric flagellate found in the small intestine. Clinical disease is more likely to occur in young animals or animals that are stressed (Hsu 1979). Necropsy of an animal with an acute infection typically reveals the presence of frothy contents in the lumen of the distended intestine (Harkness and Wagner 1983). Control depends on good sanitation practices. Treatment with nitrofurantoin or oxytetracycline has proved ineffective (Hsu 1979).

Coccidia

Eimeria nieschulzi may cause diarrhea and death in young animals. Control depends primarily on good sanitation (Hsu 1979).

Rickettsial Parasites

Hemobartonella muris infections in rats are almost always inapparent unless an animal is splenectomized or splenic function is otherwise impaired. In the latent state, organisms are not seen in peripheral blood; however, following splenectomy an active parasitemia develops, leading to a hemolytic anemia, reticulocytosis and frequently hemoglobinuria and death (Cassell et al. 1979).

Lice

Polyplax spinulosa is a blood sucking louse that causes skin irritation, anemia, and debilitation. Dusts such as malathion (3-5%), rotenone (0.5-1%), and lindane (0.25-0.5%) applied to the animals and the bedding are effective against lice. Sprays or dips, including diazinon (0.03-0.06%) and malathion (0.1-0.25%) are also effective in eliminating lice (Hsu 1979). Resin strips containing dichlorvos placed near the cage will reduce the ectoparasite population (Harkness and Wagner 1977).

Mites

Notoedres muris burrows into the deeper layers of the epidermis, producing red papules or reddened and thickened skin (Hsu 1979). Mite infestations are effectively treated by topical application of lindane solution (0.1-0.25%) and various other miticidal preparations.

Mycotic Diseases

Dermatophytosis (ringworm) in rats is usually caused by *Trichophyton mentagrophytes*. Infection may cause widespread skin lesions in a colony or may produce lesionless carriers. The effectiveness of griseofulvin for treating ringworm has not been evaluated in rats (Weisbroth 1979).

Systemic mycoses are extremely rare in rats (Weisbroth 1979).

MISCELLANEOUS CONDITIONS

Ringtail

Ringtail appears as one or more annular constrictions of the tail. Distal to the constriction, the tail may become edematous or necrotic. If the tail is sloughed, the stump will usually heal without complication.

The condition usually occurs in unweaned rats at 7-15 days of age. It is caused by housing young rats at low (20% or less) ambient relative humidity. Ringtail occurs primarily in the winter months when heating systems are in use.

Ringtail can be prevented by providing solid-bottomed cages with adequate bedding and maintaining the relative humidity at approximately 50%. Ringtail is rarely seen except in young rats housed in suspended wire cages in a room with high air turnover or in cages with hygroscopic bedding.

Chromodacryorrhea

The harderian gland in the rat orbit secretes porphyrins. When secretion becomes excessive, red tears containing porphyrin run down the nasolacrimal duct and form a red crust around the eyes and nose (Williams 1976). This reddish material resembles blood. The amount of secretion increases with age and various forms of stress such as shipping. Old rats with advanced chronic murine pneumonia may have obvious signs of chromodacryorrhea. It also may be seen in rats with sialodacryoadenitis. Treatment specifically for chromodacryorrhea is not indicated; however, the presence of excess secretions may suggest the possibility of some other underlying disease.

Adynamic Ileus

The intraperitoneal administration of high concentrations of chloral hydrate may result in adynamic ileus. Affected animals exhibit abdominal distention and lethargy prior to death (Russell et al. 1981).

Disease of Aging

A number of disease processes are commonly found in aged rats. Among the more frequently seen lesions are those of chronic renal disease, spinal nerve root degeneration, skeletal muscle degeneration, and polyarteritis nodosa (Anver and Cohen 1979).

NEOPLASMS

Mammary tumors are very common in most stocks of laboratory rats. Because of the distribution of mammary tissue, the tumors may occur over a wide area of the body and may reach enormous sizes. In rats, mammary tumors are usually classified as fibroadenomas. Most tumors are well encapsulated and do not metastasize. In a pet rat, surgical removal is feasible and prospects of recovery are favorable.

Spontaneous neoplasms involving essentially every organ have been reported, with the incidence depending to a large extent on the particular stock or strain and age of animals examined.

CHAPTER 3

MONGOLIAN GERBILS

CHARACTERISTICS

The Mongolian gerbil (Meriones unguiculatus) is also called a jird or sand rat. This rodent is a native of the desert regions of China and Mongolia. Gerbils are intermediate in size between mice and hamsters; mature animals usually weigh less than 100 g. The color of the gerbil is typically agouti, which is a sandy brown color. The tail is furred and may have a black tuft at the end.

Uses

Gerbils have several favorable attributes as pets: they are clean, friendly, and fairly quiet; leave little odor; rarely bite; and are easily handled. They have tremendous curiosity and are more active and therefore more interesting than some of the other species of so-called "pocket pets." Males thump with their rear legs to attract attention or express aggressiveness. They are banned as pets in California because of the possibility that they may escape and become established in the wild (Rich 1968).

Gerbils are gaining acceptance as research animals in several areas because of their susceptibility to a wide variety of viral, bacterial, and parasitic diseases and their somewhat unique physiologic and anatomic characteristics. They are used extensively in research on certain parasites, particularly filarial worms, and are of interest to neurologists because of their epileptiform seizures.

BIOLOGY

Anatomic Features

Gerbils have an ovoid, hairless ventral midline sebaceous gland. Pet owners may have concern that this porous tan area is abnormal. Ventral sebaceous glands or "pads" occur in both sexes but are most fully developed in adult males. The gerbil scent-marks its environment by rubbing the sebaceous pad over objects. Injecting testosterone increases gland size and marking activity in both sexes (Davis 1974).

The circle of Willis is incomplete; therefore, gerbils may develop cerebral ischemia following unilateral carotid ligation (Vincent et al. 1978).

The adrenal glands are large in size relative to the total body weight. They are about four times the size of the adrenal of a rat on a body weight basis (Davis 1974).

Basophilic stippling of some of the red blood cells is quite pronounced This is a physiologic phenomenon and not a disease and should not be confused with Eperythrozoon sp. infection (Williams 1976).

Young males have a dark scrotum, and the anogenital distance is greater in males than in females. In some cases, young gerbils may be difficult to sex because in a few animals the differences are not pronounced. The dark-colored scrotum is most obvious in recently weaned stock.

Physiology

See App. 2 for a list of normal physiologic values. Some of the more significant features follow.

Gerbils usually live from 2 to 3 yr but the life span may exceed 4 yr.

The average body temperature is 99.4°F. Gerbils tolerate a wide range of ambient temperatures; environmental temperatures ranging from below freezing to over 100°F apparently have no adverse effects.

The nephron of the gerbil is remarkably adapted to conserve water and electrolytes (Harkness and Wagner 1977). Gerbils therefore require only small quantities of water. They excrete only a few drops of concentrated urine per day, and their fecal boluses are nearly desiccated if water is restricted. This characteristic is less marked if they have free access to water.

When the relative humidity exceeds 50%, the body fur of gerbils stands out and appears matted and greasy instead of lying smoothly against the body (Williams 1976).

Even on normal diets, gerbils have high serum cholesterol levels. Despite this, gerbils are very resistant to development of arteriosclerosis (Davis 1974).

Reproduction

Puberty occurs at around 10 wk of age, which is later than other rodents commonly used in research. Gerbils are polyestrus; when light cycles are controlled to provide 12-14 hr light/day, they will usually breed throughout the year (Marston 1976). The estrus cycle is 4-6 days in length. A female in estrus acts restless and may have a congested vulva. The behavior of the two sexes is a better guide to the presence of estrus than vaginal smears. The vaginal epithelium is not a reliable indicator of the stages of the estrus cycle (Marston and Chang 1965). Ovulation is spontaneous in gerbils.

The gestation period is usually 24-26 days. Implantation may be delayed if the female is bred while suckling a large litter. Under these circumstances, the gestation period may be as long as 42 days (Marston 1976).

Pairs should be formed at 8 wk of age or earlier and should not be separated unless the pair proves to be incompatible. Breeding pairs are usually monogamous for life. A mature animal that has lost its mate will generally not accept another. Mating usually, but not always, occurs late in the evening.

A copulation plug is formed during mating, but it is small and lies deep in the vagina so that it is not readily detected.

Gerbils are not as prolific as mice and are inclined to periods of nonbreeding. Providing tin cans for hideaways, changing the bedding type, or housing in an opaque cage (Harkness and Wagner 1977) may encourage gerbils to resume breeding. Prior to weaning 30% mortality due to maternal neglect or other causes is not unusual.

The average litter size is 4-6. Smaller litters may be destroyed by the mother (Harkness and Wagner 1977). Hand rearing of orphans is not practical or usually successful.

HUSBANDRY

Housing

Gerbils that are paired or housed together in groups after reaching puberty or reunited after prolonged separation tend to fight. Techniques to avoid or reduce this tendency include (1) forming pairs or groups of gerbils at weaning or at least before they reach puberty (10 wk of age), (2) anesthetizing the animals and allowing them to recover simultaneously in a neutral cage (Harkness and Wagner 1977), and (3) placing tin cans in the cage as hiding places for subordinate animals.

Gerbils are usually caged in plastic or metal rat or mouse cages with solid bottoms. They can also be kept in glass aquariums. The enclosure should be at least 6 in. high to provide the animals adequate space to sit upright.

Wood shavings, sawdust, sand, ground corncobs, and various other products are satisfactory for bedding; however, the use of pine shavings may result in greasy-appearing, matted fur (Rich 1968). Bedding should be 1-2 in. deep to permit burrowing. Because of the small volume of urine produced, cages in a laboratory do not ordinarily require cleaning more often than every 1-2 wk. More frequent changes of bedding are desirable when gerbils are kept in the home as pets, particularly if several animals are housed together.

Nutrition

The recommended diet for gerbils is pelleted rodent chow fed ad libitum. Although gerbils prefer sunflower seeds to pelleted chows, these are not satisfactory as a total diet because sunflower seeds have a low calcium and high fat content and do not meet total nutritional needs (Harkness and Wagner 1977). Seeds should therefore be given only as a treat and not as the primary diet. A limited amount of green food such as lettuce, spinach, or carrots (which can be eaten in 10-15 min) may also be fed, although the necessity for this practice is doubtful.

Caged gerbils should be supplied continuously with clean water. In their natural state they obtain sufficient water from seeds and roots, but dry laboratory chow alone does not provide an adequate amount. The average water intake, when gerbils are fed a pelleted diet, is about 4-5 ml/100 g body weight per day, but they can maintain body weight on as little as 2 ml/100 g body weight (Arrington and Ammerman 1969). Gerbils may survive for 45 days or longer without water if not stressed, but they do not breed under these conditions (Marston 1976).

TECHNIQUES

Handling and Restraint

A gerbil may be lifted by grasping at the base of the tail, but this method should be used with caution because the skin may slip off to expose the vertebrae if the tail is handled too roughly or grasped too near the free end.

A gerbil may be restrained by first holding the tail with one hand then grasping the scruff of the neck or gripping over the back with the other hand. Although not inclined to bite, they are quick and capable of leaping great distances in an effort to escape. Gerbils tend to struggle when placed on their back; thus injections or manipulations are more readily accomplished when animals are not held in this position.

Blood Collection and Medication

Blood samples are best obtained from the orbital sinus or by heart puncture in a lightly anesthetized animal; however, neither of these techniques are acceptable in the presence of an owner. The best method for collecting blood with an owner present is to clip a toenail very short.

Up to 1/10 ml liquid medication can be administered by using a dropper at the diastema. For larger amounts a stomach tube can be passed with the animal lightly anesthetized, or a ball-ended dosing needle can be used.

Anesthesia

Anesthetic agents and suggested dosages are listed in section C.4 of App. 1.

General anesthesia lasting for 2-3 hr can be obtained with pentobarbital (Rx: C.4.c). Accuracy of dosage can be increased by diluting 1:10. A combination of ketamine and supplemental methoxyflurane using a nose cone gives simple, safe surgical anesthesia (Rx: C.4.b). Animals can also be placed in a glass container with methoxyflurane applied to cotton or gauze to induce anesthesia. Ketamine alone (Rx: C.4.a) produces sedation but does not provide good muscle relaxation; at higher dose levels recovery is prolonged, requiring 2 hr or longer. Gerbils are not good subjects for ether anesthesia (Marston 1976); nevertheless, it is used at times.

BACTERIAL DISEASES

Tyzzer's Disease

Tyzzer's disease (*Bacillus piliformis*) is the only fatal infectious disease commonly seen in gerbils. Affected animals show a roughened hair coat, lethargy, and anorexia. Diarrhea may be absent or mild in gerbils, in contrast to mice and rabbits where a profuse diarrhea is characteristic (Port et al. 1970). The disease is most frequently seen at weaning age. The mortality rate is high in young animals (3-7 wk of age) and postpartum females but low in other adults.

The characteristic lesion of Tyzzer's disease in gerbils, as in other species, is an enlarged liver with numerous gray and yellow foci 1-2 mm in diameter (Carter et al. 1969). In addition, there may be edema and hemorrhage of the intestines, particularly in the area of the ileocecal junction. Microscopically, special stains reveal the presence of filamentous microorganisms adjacent to the areas of necrosis in the liver.

Oxytetracycline (Rx: C.1.c) added to the drinking water is sometimes beneficial. Fluid therapy can be provided, if indicated, by subcutaneous injection of 4-5 ml isotonic saline solution (Clifford 1973). Outbreaks usually subside after a certain number of deaths, and the value of antibiotic treatment is questionable. Improvements in management practices, particularly the level of sanitation, are usually more rewarding than medical treatment in reducing losses (Clifford 1973).

Staphylococcal and Streptococcal Infections

Animals with abrasions or bald noses often acquire staphylococcal or streptococcal infections. Lesions typically begin around the external nares and spread to the feet, legs, and ventral surface of the body. An acute, diffuse moist dermatitis caused by *Staphylococcus aureus* may also develop in the absence of a bald nose (Peckham et al. 1974). The presence of bite wounds increase the severity of the infection.

A topical nitrofurazone ointment or other antibacterial preparation applied daily is often beneficial. For parenteral treatment, chloramphenicol (Rx: C.1.a) in the drinking water for 2 wk is recommended. With treatment, regression of clinical signs usually occurs, but recovery is not always complete and recurrence after apparent recovery is not unusual.

Salmonellosis

Gerbils are relatively resistant to *Salmonella* spp. infections. The usual response of the gerbil to *S. typhimurium* is a mild to severe diarrhea followed by complete recovery. A carrier state apparently does not exist (Schwentker 1963).

Leptospirosis

Spontaneous leptospirosis has not been reported in gerbils; however, following experimental infection with *Leptospira pomona* they remain asymptomatic but eliminate large numbers of microorganisms in the urine for a long period (Lewis and Gray 1961). Gerbils are therefore potential transmitters of leptospirosis.

PARASITIC DISEASES

Demodectic Mange

Alopecia and dermatitis associated with *Demodex* spp. have been reported in gerbils (Clifford 1973; Schwarzbrott *et al.* 1974). Goodwinol ointment is a suggested treatment (Russell et al. 1981). The ronnel-propylene glycol preparation (Rx: D.2.e) used in treating demodectic mange in hamsters may also be effective in gerbils (Harkness and Wagner 1977).

Pinworms

Pinworm infections (*Syphacia obvelata*) occur in gerbils (Ross et al. 1980; Wightman et *al. 1978*). Piperazine (Rx: C.2.a) is the drug of choice for treatment of pinworms.

Tapeworms

Gerbils are susceptible to infection by tapeworms (*Hymenolepis diminuta* and *H. nana*). Niclosamide (Rx: C.2.b) administered as a drench is recommended for treatment of tapeworms. Treatment should be repeated in 2 wk.

MISCELLANEOUS CONDITIONS

Antibiotic Toxicity

Gerbils do not develop the fatal gram-negative enterotoxemia associated with penicillin and other antibiotics having similar action in hamsters and guinea pigs; however, streptomycin has a direct toxic action. A 50-mg dose of dihydrostreptomycin will kill most gerbils within 2 hr (Wightman et al. 1980).

Biting and Chewing Vices

Gerbils may react to overcrowding by biting each other near the base of the tail, causing denuded small spots in this location. Also, animals that are bored may practice tail chewing, causing loss of hair along the tail (Williams 1976).

Bald Nose

A bald nose may result from excessive digging with the nose or pushing it through the cage bars (Williams 1976). Putting the animal in a smooth-sided box or aquarium with soft bedding and without cage bars is usually helpful.

Sebaceous Gland Disease

Midventral sebaceous glands may become infected and abscessed, usually appearing as areas of ulcerated bleeding dermatitis (Vincent et al. 1979). They also may become neoplastic; the tumors most frequently are sebaceous gland adenomas. Other tumor types involving the sebaceous gland include basal cell and squamous cell carcinomas. Local debridement and topical antibiotic or combination antibiotic-glucocorticoid-proteolytic enzyme ointments are used in treatment of abscesses. Tumors are surgically removed with wide excision (Burke 1979).

Dental Disease

Overgrowth of incisors can be corrected by trimming the teeth. Spontaneous periodontal destruction related to accumulation of plaque and calculuslike accretions has been reported in gerbils fed a commercial laboratory diet (Moskow et al. 1968) but has not been recognized as a significant clinical problem.

Chromodacryorrhea

The harderian gland in the orbit produces porphyrin. In cases of excessive secretion, a red crust will appear in the inner canthus of the eye or on the end of the nose and is often mistaken for dried blood. No treatment is indicated (Williams 1976).

Epileptiform Seizures

Epileptiform seizures may take the form of convulsions, or affected animals may enter a hypnotic or cataleptoid state. The attacks are usually initiated by some form of stress or fright, such as handling, environmental disturbances, or a novel environment. The convulsions usually last about a minute or less and are not fatal. No treatment is necessary; however, the seizure can be eliminated with drugs such as dilantin or reserpine (Russell et al. 1981). This trait has a genetic basis, and selective breeding can increase or decrease the tendency (Williams 1976).

Neoplasms and Cysts

In addition to neoplasms of the midventral sebaceous gland, other spontaneous tumors most frequently involving skin, ovary, testicle, adrenal gland, and, cecum have been observed in gerbils (Vincent and Ash 1978). Most reports indicate that neoplasms occur primarily in aged gerbils and that the incidence of ovarian tumors is high (Meckley and Zwicker 1979). Cystic ovaries are also very common in females over 2 yr of age. They range from 1 to 50 mm in diameter (Norris and Adams 1972).

CHAPTER 4

SYRIAN HAMSTERS

CHARACTERISTICS

Several species of hamster exist in various parts of the world, but only two are found in any significant number in the United States. These are the golden or Syrian hamster (*Mesocricetus auratus*) and the Chinese or striped hamster (*Cricetulus griseus*). Syrian hamsters are by far the more popular, both for research and as pets. Although called the golden hamster, they also occur in a variety of other colors, including agouti, cinnamon, cream, white, piebald, and a long-haired variety called "teddy bear." Information presented here refers primarily to the Syrian hamster.

Uses

If hamsters are handled gently and often, they usually become docile pets; however, if roughly handled or startled, they frequently bite. Hamsters are adept at chewing on and escaping from their cages (Harkness and Wagner 1977).

Hamsters are important and popular research animals. They have proven valuable in a number of areas of biomedical research particularly in studies of cancer, infectious disease , and hypothermia. Hamsters are also used in research involving dental caries and tissue response to dental materials.

BIOLOGY

Anatomic Features

Hamsters have well-developed cheek pouches in which they transport and store food. These pouches are devoid of glands, are highly distensible, and appear to be immunologically privileged sites. They can be pulled with forceps from an anesthetized animal's mouth for examination or manipulation.

The adult male posseses two well-developed hip glands that are dark pigmented spots with roughened skin and coarse, darkly colored hair in the flank region. The intensity of the pigmentation is an indication of sex hormone activity. When the male becomes sexually excited, the fur above the gland becomes wet and he scratches and rubs this spot (Clark 1975a). It is thought that the hip glands are used for olfactory identification of territory (Magalhaes 1968). In the female the glands are poorly developed and scarcely visible.

Two large fat bodies are located immediately cranial to the testes.

Hamster kidneys are remarkable for the extremely long papillae that extend into the ureter; they make possible the collection of urine samples from single collecting tubules in living animals (Magalhaes 1968).

Differentiation between adult males and females is rather simple and can be determined without handling the animal. When viewed from above, the perineal margin of the male hamster is rounded due to the scrotal sac; the female has a blunt rear end. Sexual differentiation requires closer examination in younger animals; the distance from the external urethral orifice to the anus is greater in males than females. In addition, testicles can usually be seen in young males.

Physiology

Normal physiologic data are listed in App. 2.

The normal rectal temperature of a hamster is betwen 98 and 100°F.

The usual life span is from 18 to 24 mo, with occasional animals living 3-4 yr.

REPRODUCTION

Golden hamsters are usually bred for the first time at 6-8 wk of age at a weight of 80-100 g (Harkness and Wagner 1977).

Except for the period of estrus, the female will usually attack a newly introduced male. At the onset of estrus the female becomes nonbelligerent toward the male and secretes a vaginal discharge. On day 1 there may be a slight translucent discharge; mating usually occurs on the evening of day 1, 1-2 hr after dark. On day 2 a copious postovulatory discharge with a gray-white color and a distinctive odor is secreted. Pregnancy can be confirmed in hamsters by examining for a postovulatory discharge on days 5 and 9 after mating. If the female has a postovulatory discharge at these times, she is not pregnant but is having normal estrus cycles (Clark 1975b). When a female in estrus is placed with a male, a short getting-acquainted period occurs; then the female arches her back downward in a position of lordosis and repeated intromissions and ejaculations occur during a period of 20-60 min (Clark 1975b).

The gestation period of a hamster ranges from 15 to 18 days with a 16-day average, and the young are weaned at 3 wk of age.

Behavior

Adult hamsters, particularly females, usually should be caged individually because of their tendency to fight. Groups formed before reaching sexual maturity are less inclined to fight than adult animals placed together (Harkness and Wagner 1977).

Cannibalism of the young is quite common, particularly during the first week of life (Clark 1975b). To reduce this risk, the young should not be handled for at least 5 days postpartum, especially if the female hamster is primiparous. At 14 days after mating, the female should be placed in a clean cage with clean bedding, food, and nesting material. For the next 7 to 10 days, the mother and young should be disturbed as little as possible. The addition of bits of apple or lettuce to the diet prior to parturition is also advocated by some as a means of preventing cannibalism (Williams 1976).

Fostering is rarely successful. Neonatal hamsters are immature and hand rearing is extremely difficult if not impossible (Harkness and Wagner 1977).

Conditions of low light intensity, short day length, quietness, and cool temperature induce hibernation. The hamster is considered a "permissive hibernator" because it can, to an extent, determine whether or not it will enter a state of hibernation (Hoffman 1968). If housed together, not all animals in a box will necessarily hibernate at the same time, and the active ones may cannibalize the sleepers (Williams 1976).

Medication

Hamsters exhibit a unique response to some drugs, and clinical veterinarian should be aware of these idiosyncrasies.

They are extremely resistant to the effects of morphine (Wills 1968).

They have a greater tolerance for pentobarbital than most other laboratory animals, and higher doses are required to produce anesthesia.

Penicillin, erythromycin, lincomycin, and various other antibiotics are often lethal to hamsters. These antibiotics cause death by eliminating the gram-positive intestinal flora, thus leading to a fatal gram-negative enterotoxemia with death occurring several days after administration. A toxin produced by *Clostridium difficile* appears to cause enterocolitis and death following administration of these antibiotics (Bartlett et al. 1978). Dihydrostreptomycin, on the other hand, is directly toxic and will kill hamsters in less than an hour.

HUSBANDRY

Housing

Caging used for other laboratory rodents is satisfactory for hamsters.

Nutrition

Hamsters do well on commercial pelleted diets manufactured for rats and mice. Young hamsters will begin eating solid dry food at about 7-10 days of age. Water should be available when they begin to consume dry food, or gastrointestinal disturbances will result (Clark 1975b).

TECHNIQUES

Handling and Restraint

Before handling a hamster, it is important to make sure that it is awake and expects to be picked up. Startled or suddenly awakened hamsters often bite. A number of methods are used for holding or lifting a hamster. Hamsters can be moved from one cage to another by placing both hands under the animal, palms upward, and bringing them up around the animal like a scoop or by putting a tin can in the cage, which the hamster will enter. A hamster may be restrained by picking it up by the loose skin at the scruff of the neck or over the back or may be grasped by simply placing a hand around the thorax.

Blood Collection

Small amounts of blood can be obtained from the orbital sinus, by severing the tip of the tail, or by making a slit in the foot pad. A larger volume is most readily collected by means of a heart puncture.

Drug Administration

The femoral or saphenous vein is used for intravenous injections.

Drugs that do not have an unpleasant taste can be added to the drinking water.

Anesthesia

Anesthetic dosages are listed in section D.3 of App. 1.

Premedication with 44 mg/kg ketamine followed by methoxyflurane administered with a nose cone (Rx: D.3.d) is one of the safest and most satisfactory methods of producing surgical anesthesia in hamsters. Although ether is sometimes used, it is irritating to mucous membranes.

BACTERIAL DISEASES

Proliferative Ileitis

Hamsters are susceptible to many experimentally induced infections; however, spontaneous systemic infections other than proliferative enteritis are relatively rare. This disease, also called transmissible ileal hyperplasia, wet tail, or regional enteritis, is the most important and devastating of hamster diseases. The specific etiology is not entirely certain; but growing evidence indicates that *Campylobacter* spp. and *Escherichia coli* are the primary pathogens, with each accounting for different features of the syndrome (Harkness and Wagner 1977; Lentsch et al. 1982). Clinical disease usually occurs at 3 to 8 wk of age. Stress plays an important role in susceptibility to clinical disease, with improper diet, transportation, crowding, and poor sanitation significant predisposing factors. Typical clinical signs of proliferative enteritis are diarrhea, a moistened perianal area, and high mortality (often 90% of the affected animals will die). Anorexia and a ruffled hair coat are nonspecific signs usually observed. Sometimes a hamster may have a watery diarrhea, while at other times the fecal pellets appear normal, but as they are passed, watery fluid is expelled simultaneously (Williams 1976). Death usually occurs within 1-7 days after onset of clinical signs. Animals surviving the acute disease often develop strictures, diverticula, multifocal hepatic abscesses, and adhesions (Harkness and Wagner 1977).

The disease primarily affects the ileum and terminal jejunum. This segment of intestine is congested and often ulcerated and contains yellow fluid. Marked enlargement of the ileum resulting from thickening of the mucosa is a characteristic lesion except in animals that die very acutely. Microscopically, epithelial hyperplasia of the mucosa is evident, and regenerating glands may extend into the submucosa and subserosa. At one time, the lesion was regarded by some as an adenocarcinoma.

Neomycin (Rx: D.1.e) administered for 3-5 days is the most popular drug for treating wet tail. Animals may be dosed individually or by adding the antibiotic to the drinking water. Neomycin has also been used successfully in the prevention of disease (Sheffield and Beveridge 1962). Tetracycline (Rx: D.1.f) and gentamicin (Rx: D.1.d) have also been used successfully. To be effective, antibiotics must be administered early in the course of the disease, and even then results are often disappointing. Supportive therapy with whole milk or buttermilk is reported to be beneficial in some cases (Russell et al. 1981) as has an increase in room temperature (Sebesteny 1979). Fluid administration should be considered if the sentimental value of the animal justifies the cost. The importance of correcting any management problems and eliminating stress factors should not be overlooked.

Miscellaneous Bacterial Diseases

Streptococcus spp. and *Pasteurella pneumotropica* infections may cause pneumonia. The illness is usually acute with affected animals exhibiting an ocular discharge and wheezing (Russell et al 1981). Tetracycline (Rx: D.1.f), gentamicin (Rx: D.1.d), and chloramphenicol (Rx: D.1.b) are useful in treating bacterial pneumonia in hamsters. Any adverse environmental conditions that may exist should be corrected.

Salmonella spp. infections usually produce an acute septicemic or enteric disease with a high mortality. The lesions are similar to those seen with salmonellosis in other rodent species (McClure et al. 1978).

Staphylococcus aureus may cause abscesses and arthritis (Russell et al. 1981).

Tyzzer's disease (*Bacillus piliformis*) may cause death with few premonitory signs or diarrhea, lethargy, and anorexia may be evident, with death usually within 1-3 days after onset of clinical signs (Carlton and Hunt 1978). Tetracycline (Rx: D.1.f) is sometimes beneficial in treating this disease. Although the risk of antibiotic toxicity is increased by using a greater than usual dosage for treating bacterial infections in hamsters, the practice may improve effectiveness of tetracycline.

Yersinia pseudotuberculosis infections are uncommon in hamsters. The disease usually follows a chronic course and is characterized by formation of caseous nodules in the mesenteric lymph nodes, spleen, liver, and lungs (Russell et al. 1981).

VIRAL DISEASES

Lymphocytic Choriomeningitis

In 1974 the occurrence of several cases of human lymphocytic choriomeningitis contracted from pet hamsters was widely publicized (Williams 1976). However, hamsters are one of many species susceptible to infection with lymphocytic choriomeningitis virus and are regarded as less likely sources of human infection than mice.

Other Viral Infections

Hamsters are susceptible to infection by a number of murine viruses, but clinical disease from natural infection is rarely recognized.

PARASITIC DISEASES

Mites

Demodex creceti is a short, stubby-bodied mite. Some authors do not consider this species to be pathogenic, (Williams 1976) while others state that the mite causes epidermal damage and alopecia (Flynn 1973). *D. aurati* has the cigar-shaped body typical of a demodectic mange mite and burrows into the skin, producing hyperpigmentation, a dry scaly dermatitis, and alopecia (Flynn 1973). These mites are quite common in pet hamsters.

Demodectic mange can be treated with various miticidal creams or lotions. A mixture or ronnel concentrate and propylene glycol is suggested as treatment (Rx: D.2.e). The preparation may be applied to one-third of the body daily until skin scrapings are negative (Burke 1979).

Pinworms

Syphacia obvelata occurs in hamsters but rarely if ever causes clinical disease (Williams 1976). Piperazine (Rx: D.2.c) is effective in treating pinworms.

Tapeworms

Heavy infections with *Hymenolepis nana* may cause diarrhea (Williams 1976). These tapeworms can be eliminated by administration of niclosamide (Rx: D.2.b).

Protozoa

Numerous protozoa, including *Trichomonas* sp., *Hexamita* sp., and *Giardia* sp., are harbored in the intestines but are of no clinical significance (Williams 1976).

MISCELLANEOUS CONDITIONS

Overgrown Incisors

In determining the cause for refusal to eat, the mouth should be carefully examined. A hamster may be unable to eat because of overgrown incisor teeth. Bone cutters or a rotary cutting tool may be used to shorten overgrown incisors.

Impacted Cheek Pouches

Hamsters will sometimes overload their cheek pouches. Affected animals will have large swellings on one or both sides of the face or shoulder. The pouches should be emptied with forceps and flushed with a syringe and plain water. An antibiotic ointment may be applied if abrasion of the cheek pouch is severe.

Cage Paralysis

A nutritional myopathy caused by a deficiency of vitamin D or E may occur in hamsters when the diet is limited to table scraps, but it is unlikely to develop in animals receiving commercial rodent chows. Stiffness from lack of exercise can be corrected by providing an exercise wheel. Paralysis is most frequently the result of injuries sustained when animals are dropped onto a hard surface.

Trauma

As with other small rodents, external splinting is often not satisfactory. Stainless steel hypodermic needles used as intramedullary pins for fracture repair may be preferable to external fixation for repair of fractured long bones.

Fine stainless steel wire is preferable to other material for suturing lacerations, because it is not gnawed out so quickly.

Vaginitis

The opaque, white postovulatory discharge that appears at the time of estrus should not be confused with a vaginitis.

Amyloidosis

Syrian hamsters have a high incidence of amyloidosis. The disease is generalized and considered to be a primary type. Amyloid deposits begin to appear in animals under 1 yr of age and the disease progresses with the age of the animal (Casey et al. 1978).

Polycystic Disease

Polycystic disease is another condition often seen in hamsters over 1 year of age. Cysts are most frequently found in the epididymis, seminal vesicles, pancreas, and liver (Clark 1975a).

Hemorrhagic Necrosis of the Central Nervous System

A spontaneous hemorrhagic necrosis of the central nervous system in fetal hamsters has occurred in commercial production colonies on several occasions. The etiology of this disease is uncertain; however, the problem is reported to be preventable by high vitamin E supplementation during gestation and lactation (Keeler and Young 1979).

CHAPTER 5

GUINEA PIGS

CHARACTERISTICS

Taxonomy

The scientific name of the guinea pig is *Cavia porcellus*. Guinea pigs are hystricomorph rodents originating from South America. They are more closely related to porcupines and chinchillas than to mice or rats (Clark and Baker 1975b).

Genetic Types

The English, Abyssinian, and Peruvian varieties (Clark and Baker 1975b) are the three major types of guinea pigs in the United States; they can be distinguished by the length, texture, and direction of hair growth. English guinea pigs have short, smooth, straight, coarse hair. There are a number of outbred and inbred strains of English guinea pigs, and most guinea pigs used in research are of this type. Abyssinian guinea pigs have short coarse hair arranged in whorls, which gives them an untidy appearance. Peruvian guinea pigs have long, fine, silky hair.

Uses

The docile nature of guinea pigs accounts for their popularity as pets. They seldom bite or scratch and will respond to attention with frequent and gentle handling. On the other hand, they tend to be messy, and the development of human allergies to guinea pigs is not uncommon.

Guinea pigs, though perhaps not used in the numbers perceived by the general public, are important research animals that are used primarily in studies of immunology, audiology, and infectious disease (Clark and Baker 1975b). They are relatively expensive, usually costing three to five times as much as rats and often as much as rabbits; however, perhaps their greatest disadvantage for research use is the lack of readily accessible peripheral veins for injections and blood collection.

BIOLOGY

Anatomic Features

The incisor and cheek teeth of guinea pigs are open rooted and grow continuously throughout life. Between the incisors and cheek teeth is a gap, the diastema.

Kurloff bodies are eosinophilic intracytoplasmic inclusion bodies found in mononuclear leukocytes in the circulating blood, spleen, thymus, bone marrow, and placenta. These are more numerous in females than in males and tend to increase in number during pregnancy and after estrogen administration (Clark and Baker 1975a).

Guinea pig neutrophils, like those of rabbits, have red granules in the cytoplasm (Williams 1976).

Perivascular lymphoid nodules are frequently found in the lungs of guinea pigs. They tend to occur around the smaller branches of the pulmonary arteries and veins (Wagner 1976). Their significance is uncertain at this time.

Guinea pigs have one pair of mammary glands in the inguinal region. Other rodents such as mice and rats have several pairs of mammary glands.

The genital region of the female guinea pig has a Y-shaped crease; in the male the structure is seen as more of a straight slit, which is a fold between the two halves of the scrotum. The difference in appearance of the external genitalia may not be readily apparent to the inexperienced observer, and palpation or extrusion of the penis by gentle digital pressure may be necessary to establish the sex.

Physiology

Normal physiologic data are listed in App. 2.

The usual life span of guinea pigs is 5-6 yr.

Reproduction

Puberty can occur as early as 3 or 4 wk of age in females, however, they are not ordinarily bred at this age. Normally, males are used as breeders at the age of 4-5 mo (weighing about 550 g) and females at 3-5 mo of age (weighing about 500 g) (Harkness and Wagner 1977). The gestation period may range from 59 to 72 days but generally is from 63 to 68 days. The length of the gestation period depends primarily on the number of fetuses in the litter; litters of fewer fetuses have a longer gestation period (Harkness and Wagner 1977) and a greater individual birth weight. A guinea pig is more completely developed at birth than any other familiar species of laboratory animal. They are fully furred and can consume solid food within a few hours of birth (Clark 1975a). The young are generally weaned at 2-3 wk of age.

HUSBANDRY

Housing

Since guinea pigs are not inclined to climb, they can be kept in open-top boxes provided the sides are at least 10 in. high. Grid or mesh floors facilitate cage cleaning; however, solid floors with bedding are preferred for breeding animals. The room temperature should be maintained between 65 and 75°F. They are quite sensitive to temperature extremes but tolerate low temperatures better than high temperatures (Clark and Baker 1975b).

Nutrition

Guinea pigs and nonhuman primates are the only common species of laboratory animals that require a dietary source of vitamin C. Commercial guinea pig chows are fortified with this vitamin. If uncertain about the freshness of the diet, guinea pigs can be fed green vegetables such as cabbage or kale. The risk of contamination can be avoided by adding about 200 mg/L ascorbic acid to the drinking water rather than feeding green vegetables (Harkness and Wagner 1977). Water fortified with ascorbic acid should be provided in glass or plastic bottles rather than in metal containers or open bowls to prolong the activity of the added vitamins. The use of distilled or deionized water rather than chlorinated tap water will also reduce the rate of vitamic C deactivation (Clark and Baker 1975b).

Some sources advocate feeding good quality hay such as alfalfa. Some nutritional benefit may be derived from the hay and it also provides roughage. Probably the most important benefit, however, is to provide a diversion for the animals and reduce the incidence of chewing the hair of either their cage mates or themselves.

TECHNIQUES

Handling

Guinea pigs should be lifted by grasping the trunk with one hand while supporting the rear quarters with the other. Support is particularly important with adults and pregnant animals. Injured lungs may result if an animal is grasped too firmly over its back.

Blood Collection

Guinea pigs lack readily accessible peripheral veins. Small amounts of blood can be collected from the orbital sinus or by clipping a toenail. Larger amounts of blood can be obtained from the femoral artery or vein or directly from the heart. Cardiac puncture is best carried out with the animal lightly anesthetized. The guinea pig can either be placed on its right side and the needle inserted at the site of the apex beat around the fourth intercostal space or on its back and the needle inserted in the zyphoid area, aiming for the left ventricle. Cardiac punctures involve a significant element of risk.

Drug Administration

Although requiring a steady hand and a degree of skill, intravenous injections can be made using either the saphenous vein or the dorsolateral vein of the penis. A cut-down may be required for exposure of the saphenous vein. Guinea pig skin is tough, especially over the back, and subcutaneous injections require a degree of force.

Liquids can be administered orally by inserting a tuberculin syringe or a ball-ended dosing needle into the mouth through the diastema. Palatable drugs can be incorporated into the food or water, but guinea pigs will often refuse food or water with an unfamiliar taste.

Anesthesia

Guinea pigs are generally considered poor risks for anesthesia. At times they may exhibit a peculiar squirming movement during administration of volatile anesthetics. This movement does not signify return to consciousness, and caution should be exercised in administering additional anesthetic (Clark 1975a). Some of the commonly used anesthetic agents and recommended dosages are listed in section E.4 of App. 1.

Methoxyflurane is probably the safest and most satisfactory general anesthetic agent for guinea pigs. A preanesthetic administered by injection may be used to facilitate induction, and surgical anesthesia may be maintained using methyoxyflurane. Ketamine produces sedation but by itself does not produce sufficient muscular relaxation for major surgery. Good results are achieved by the combination of ketamine with methoxyflurane or various other agents. Innovar-vet produces good anesthesia; however, when used at high dosage levels, a delayed self-mutilation of the injected leg may occur following its administration. A significant degree of risk exists in using barbiturates for general anesthesia, largely because intraperitoneal injections preclude the titration of dosage to the desired depth of anesthesia. Ether in a closed jar is used for anesthesia, but experience is required to safely administer this anesthetic to guinea pigs. Because of irritation to mucous membranes by ether, guinea pigs tend to salivate excessively and hold their breath as long as possible during induction and then take a series of deep but fatal inspirations.

CASTRATION

In castrating a male guinea pig, the surgeon should incise the tunic, then grasp the testicle, and apply gentle traction to expose the spermatic cord and a mass of fat. A ligature is then placed around the cord below the mass of fat, including the tunic, before severing the cord. This technique reduces the possibility of intestinal prolapse following castration (Williams 1976).

DISEASE PREDISPOSITION AND DETECTION

Predisposing Factors

Guinea pigs are highly susceptible to factors in the environment that lower their resistance to infection. Among these are poor sanitation, overcrowding, mixing of species, improper temperature and humidity control, inadequate diet (especially insufficient vitamin C), transportation, and experimental procedures (Wagner 1979).

Detection of Illness

Illness may not be readily apparent to the inexperienced eye. A healthy guinea pig will feel dense and be tense and very alert. Lassitude and light weight are unfavorable signs (Williams 1979).

BACTERIAL DISEASES

Bacterial Pneumonia

Bacterial pneumonia is a frequent cause of death in guinea pigs. *Bordetella bronchiseptica* and *Streptococcus pneumoniae* are the organisms most often recovered in outbreaks of bacterial pneumonia. Rabbits may serve as asymptomatic carriers of *B. bronchiseptica*; and should not be housed in the same room as guinea pigs.

B. bronchiseptica and *S. pneumoniae* may exist as latent respiratory infections and clinical disease precipitated by stress. Affected animals may die acutely without obvious signs of illness or may exhibit dyspnea, nasal discharge, and other nonspecific signs such as anorexia, lassitude, and ruffled fur. Necropsy of terminal cases of *B. bronchiseptica* infection show various degrees of pulmonary consolidation and tracheitis. The trachea may contain frothy, blood-tinged exudate; the lungs may have a firm consistency and appear dark red or gray in color. A seropurulent or fibrinopurulent pleuritis, pericarditis, and peritonitis are characteristic of *S. pneumoniae* infections (Ganaway 1976).

Chloramphenicol (Rx: E.1.b, Rx: E.1.c), cephaloridine (Rx: E.1.a), tetracycline (Rx: E.1.k) and sulfamethazine (Rx: E.1.i) are among the antimicrobials most frequently used in treatment of bacterial pneumonia in guinea pigs. A killed bacterin may be used for prevention of *Bordetella bronchiseptica* infections. This is the only bacterial disease of guinea pigs for which a vaccine is available (Ganaway 1976).

Cervical Lymphadenitis

Cervical lymphadenitis, characterized by abscessation of the cervical lymph nodes, is commonly seen in guinea pigs. *Streptococcus zooepidemicus* is the usual cause; however, *Streptobacillus moniliformis* and other bacteria are occasionally incriminated. Breeders often refer to the condition as "lumps." Initially, the swollen lymph nodes are firm in consistency; but as the disease progresses, the lymphatic tissue is replaced by thick, creamy purulent exudate resulting in prominent soft swellings in the ventral cervical region of affected guinea pigs.

The infection is spread by various routes, including bite wounds and abrasion of the oral mucosa by rough food such as coarse hay. Generally the animals do not appear to be sick or particularly bothered by the abscessed lymph nodes; although sometimes an acute, fatal, septicemic disease or pneumonia may occur with a *Streptococcus zooepidemicus* infection. Occasionally, an otitis interna is caused by *S. zooepidemicus.*

Treatment ranges from a conservative approach with an appropriate antibiotic such as cephaloridine (Rx: E.1.a) for 5-7 days to surgical incision and drainage of the involved lymph nodes. If the abscesses are large and soft, the animal can be sedated with ketamine and the abscess opened, drained and flushed with 2% chlorhexidine or tincture of iodine (Harkness and Wagner 1977).

Salmonellosis

Salmonellosis is an infrequent but usually highly lethal disease of guinea pigs. The serotypes of *Salmonella* most frequently isolated from guinea pigs are *S. typhimurium* and *S. enteriditis.* The most likely source of infection in a colony is the ingestion of contaminated food, especially fresh, green leafy vegetables that have been inadequately washed before feeding (Ganaway 1976).

Salmonellosis usually occurs as an acute to subacute fatal septicemia. Clinical signs may include anorexia, weight loss, light-colored soft feces, conjunctivitis, dyspnea, and abortions. In acute cases, gross lesions may be absent at necropsy. Splenomegaly is usually seen in subacute and chronic infections, along with yellow-white nodules in the spleen, liver, and other organs. Rupture of these nodules may result in a purulent peritonitis or pleuritis (Ganaway 1976). A definitive diagnosis depends on the presence of typical lesions on histopathology and on recovery of organisms from the spleen, blood, or feces.

Treatment is usually not undertaken in case of an outbreak. The recommended approach is to kill all affected and contact animals and disinfect well.

Ulcerative Pododermatitis

Staphylococcus aureus is the usual causative agent of ulcerative pododermatitis in guinea pigs. In this condition a granuloma occurs on the ventral surface of one or more feet and may progress to osteoarthritis. It is also called "bumblefoot" and is analogous to "bumblefoot" in poultry. Ulcerative pododermatitis most frequently occurs in heavy animals held for long periods on wire mesh floors. Housing on rusted or soiled floors increases the probability of pododermatitis.

Treatment involves removing animals to a cage with clean, dry, soft bedding and administration of parenteral antibiotics, but results are often discouraging. There are seldom pus pockets to be opened and drained (Harkness and Wagner 1977).

A condition that may be confused with this lesion is one that is caused by injection of antigen plus complete Freund's adjuvant into the foot pad. This research technique is widely used by immunologists to increase the titer of antibodies against an injected antigen (Williams 1976).

Pseudotuberculosis

Infection with *Yersinia pseudotuberculosis* may exist in an acute, rapidly fatal, septicemic form; a chronic form with diarrhea and death in 3-4 wk; or a nonfatal infection with abscessed lymph nodes in the head and neck (Ganaway 1976). The disease is uncommon in guinea pigs and treatment is rarely effective.

VIRAL AND CHLAMYDIAL DISEASES

Salivary Gland Virus (Cytomegalovirus)

Cytomegalovirus infection produces large eosinophilic intranuclear inclusions in the ductal epithelium of the salivary glands of guinea pigs. The incidence of infection is very high in some colonies; however, no clinical signs or gross lesions have been associated with the virus in guinea pigs (Van Hoosier and Robinette 1976).

Cavian Leukemia

Spontaneous lymphatic leukemia of apparent viral etiology occurs in guinea pigs (Van Hoosier and Robinette 1976). Reports of incidence of the disease vary, but most indicate that it is a relatively uncommon cause of death in guinea pigs.

Lymphocytic Choriomeningitis

Lymphocytic choriomeningitis (LCM) occurs as a natural but apparently rather infrequent disease in guinea pigs. Clinical signs may be absent, or affected animals may develop a meningitis with posterior paralysis. Human infections can result from contact with LCM-infected animals (Van Hoosier and Robinette 1976).

Inclusion Body Conjunctivitis

An organism classified as a chlamydia (Psittacosis-lymphogranuloma-trachoma) produces a mild, self-limiting conjunctivitis of little clinical significance (Baker and Clark 1975). The agent is apparently enzootic in some herds and not in others (Van Hoosier and Robinette 1976).

PARASITIC DISEASES

Protozoan Parasites

The cysts of *Balantidium caviae* may be found in the feces of guinea pigs, but the organism is not considered a primary pathogen.

Coccidia affecting guinea pigs include the following:

1. *Eimeria caviae*, the intestinal coccidia of guinea pigs, is usually nonpathogenic but occasionally causes colitis, diarrhea, and death. Because the sporulation time is 6-12 days, good sanitation disrupts the life cy-

cle of the parasite (Williams 1976). Clinical disease is seldom encountered in research institutions but may occur in pet shops. Sulfonamides in the drinking water are effective if treatment is required (Rx: E.1.g; Rx: E.1.h; Rx: E.1.j).

2. *Klossiella cobayae* is a coccidium found in the renal tubules of guinea pigs. No clinical signs have been associated with infections by *K. cobayae*, and microscopic examination of tissue sections is usually required for detection of the organism (Vetterling 1976).

Pinworms

The cecal pinworm (*Paraspidodera uncinata*) is the only helminth reported from the guinea pig with any degree of frequency and it rarely causes clinical disease (Wescott 1976). With heavy infections, however, it can cause diarrhea and unthriftiness (Peters 1981). The presence of the parasite can be established by detection of eggs on fecal examination. Piperazine (Rx: E.2.d) in the drinking water is usually an effective treatment.

Lice and Fur Mites

Lice (*Gyropus ovalis* and *Gliricola porcelli*) and fur mites (*Chirodiscoides caviae*) may be found on guinea pigs. Cat flea powder (Peters 1981) or malathion dips (Rx: E.2.c) are effective against these external parasites.

Sarcoptoid Mites

The sarcoptoid mite (*Trixacarus caviae*) has been recognized in this country only recently. It causes alopecia, epidermal scaling, and intense pruritis with self-trauma. Severe infections may be fatal. The mite is often not readily detected by skin scrapings.

Suggested treatments include lime sulfur in 6 weekly baths using a 1:40 concentration (McDonald and Lavoipierre 1980), gamma benzene hexachloride applied 4 times at 10-day intervals (Russell et al. 1981), or 3 weekly applications of 1% lindane (Zajac et al. 1980).

MYCOTIC DISEASES

Superficial Mycosis

Spontaneous dermatophytosis occurs quite frequently with demonstrable lesions seen predominantly in young guinea pigs (Sprouse 1976). Superficial fungal infections (ringworm) are most commonly caused by *Trichophyton mentagrophytes*, which does not fluoresce under ultraviolet light. Lesions usually arise on the face and spread to the trunk and limbs. Clinically apparent lesions typically appear as scaly areas. If deep tissue suppuration occurs, kerions (moist, raised hairless lesions) may be formed.

Topical ointments or oral griseofulvin (Rx: E.1.d) may be used in treatment of ringworm in guinea pigs. An excellent response has been reported with use of 1 1/2% solution of griseofulvin in dimethylsulfoxide applied to lesions for 5-7 days (Post and Saunders 1979).

Systemic Mycoses

Few reports of spontaneous systemic mycotic infections are found in the literature (Sprouse 1976).

NUTRITIONAL DISEASES

Scurvy

Signs of scurvy usually appear within 2 wk after guinea pigs are deprived of vitamin C. Guinea pig diet should provide 15-20 mg vitamin C/kg body weight for maintenance (Clark and Baker 1975a); vitamin C deficiencies frequently occur when guinea pigs are fed rabbit chow. Although rabbit pellets resemble guinea pig pellets in appearance, rabbit pellets lack vitamin C, are lower in protein, and therefore do not meet the dietary requirements of guinea pigs.

Clinical signs of a vitamin C deficiency are reluctance to move, an unkempt appearance, swellings around the joints, diarrhea, and cutaneous sores. Animals often succumb to secondary bacterial infections before classical signs of scurvy are evident. The most prominent gross lesions seen at necropsy are hemorrhages in the muscle and periosteum, particularly around the stifle joint and rib cage, and epiphyseal enlargement, best noted at the costochondral junction (Harkness and Wagner 1977).

Animals showing signs of vitamin C deficiency should receive a high level of 20-50 mg/day of oral or parenteral ascorbic acid until recovery is evident. The administration of vitamin C should be considered in animals that become anorectic from any cause. Guinea pigs do not object to the flavor of ascorbic acid solution and will usually drink it from the end of a syringe (Williams 1979).

Soft Tissue Calcification

A dietary imbalance of minerals may lead to soft tissue calcification resulting in lameness and occasionally intestinal obstruction and death (Williams 1976).

Vitamin E Deficiency

Guinea pigs are very susceptible to vitamin E deficiencies, usually resulting in development of skeletal muscle necrosis, but a deficiency is unlikely in animals fed commercially produced diets (Wagner 1979).

MISCELLANEOUS CONDITIONS

Antibiotic Toxicity

Guinea pigs are highly sensitive to antibiotics, particularly those specific for gram-positive organisms. The normal intestinal flora of guinea pigs is predominantly gram-positive. Administration of antibiotics specific for gram-positive bacteria destroys the normal flora of the intestinal tract and permits an overgrowth of gram-negative organisms. Until recently, complications following antibiotic administration were attributed primarily to *E. coli*; but strong evidence now exists that *Clostridium difficile* plays an important role in the enterotoxemia that follows antibiotic treatment (Rehg and Pakes 1981). The danger is not only from parenterally administered antibiotics but also those topically applied. The antibiotics are not directly toxic and are not harmful when administered in therapeutic dosages to germ-free animals. Tetracycline, cephaloridine, chloramphenicol, and the sulfonamides are among the less hazardous antimicrobials, but all should be administered with caution, using the minimal effective dosage.

Malocclusion

Guinea pigs have open-rooted cheek teeth that grow continuously. If teeth do not properly occlude, they are not worn away and an overgrowth results. Malocclusion may be caused by genetic or dietary factors or a combination. Tooth overgrowth in guinea pigs usually involves premolars and anterior molars. Maxillary teeth grow laterally into the labial mucosa, while mandibular teeth overgrow to the lingual side (Wagner 1976). The premolar and molar teeth are difficult to examine in a conscious guinea pig because of the abundance of loose buccal skin.

Guinea pigs with cheek tooth malocclusion typically will have chronic weight loss and drool saliva ("slobbers"). The fur under the jaw and down the neck will be soaked with saliva and is sometimes stained a green or yellow color. Temporary relief can be provided by clipping or filing the teeth; however, trimming the molar teeth is difficult.

Trauma

The most commonly encountered traumatic injury in guinea pigs is fracture of the rear leg. The tibia is usually the bone involved. In research facilities where guinea pigs are often housed on wire mesh flooring, fractures may result when young pigs catch their legs in the flooring. With pet animals, the fractures often result from being dropped by children. A simple lightweight splint can be applied to provide support for the fractured bone (Williams 1976).

Ketosis (Pregnancy Toxemia)

The exact cause of pregnancy toxemia is not known but seems to involve uterine anoxia and other factors (Harkness and Wagner 1977). Obesity, sudden dietary changes, anorexia, increased fetal load, hereditary patterns, lack of exercise, sex, parity, and nonspecific environmental stressors are factors that predispose guinea pigs to ketosis. The disease is usually seen in well-nourished sows in late pregnancy but may also occur in males or virgin females. A history of change in diet or housing is a frequent feature of this disease.

Ketosis usually has an acute onset, and affected animals show signs of lethargy and severe depression. The breath typically has an acetone odor. The most prominent lesion seen at necropsy is a diffuse fatty liver. Other signs may include reduced gastric content, an abundance of body fat, near-term fetuses, uterine hemorrhage, enlarged adrenals, and tan to yellow kidneys.

The incidence can be reduced in breeding sows by controlling food intake to prevent obesity and breeding at 450-500 g body weight. Breeding sows should not be disturbed by changing diets, moving to new quarters, or other factors that might induce fasting. Ringer's solution, calcium gluconate, or dextrose (1-2 ml 50% dextrose in 3-5 ml saline) by the intravenous or intraperitoneal route in conjunction with corticosteroids can be administered as treatment, but the prognosis is poor (Williams 1976).

Experimental constriction of blood flow to the uterus will produce a syndrome very similar to preeclampsia in humans (Golden et al. 1980); the guinea pig thus may be a useful model for study of this condition in humans.

Dystocia

Approximately 5-7 days before parturition the pubic symphysis of a pregnant sow becomes separated, permitting an increased diameter of the birth canal (Sisk 1976). Sows bred for the first time at 6-9 mo of age may experience dystocia caused by fusion and ossification of the symphysis. Dystocia can also result from an excessively large fetus, obesity, and/or uterine inertia. Subclinical ketosis has been suggested as a possible factor in the etiology of some cases of dystocia (Wagner 1976).

Uterine inertia may respond to adminstration of oxytocin (Rx: E.3.c). If parturition has not begun within 15 min of oxytocin administration, cesarean section should be performed (Peters 1981).

Fetal Death

Stillbirths and abortions commonly occur in guinea pigs without obvious cause. Some authorities think that stillbirths are a common sequela of subclinical ketosis (Wagner 1976).

Alopecia

A diffuse loss of hair over the flanks and back develops to a degree in all sows in late pregnancy. It is more marked with an intensive breeding program. Around the time of weaning, a thinning of hair occurs during the transition from baby fur to more mature hair (Wagner 1976). Alopecia also seems to be associated with other stress conditions, although the exact cause is not known. Nutritional and genetic factors are probably involved to some degree.

Loss of hair with a distinctive pattern or patchy distribution can result from a hair-chewing vice termed "barbering." Animals may chew their own hair or that of a cage mate. The location of hair loss can usually provide a clue as to whether it is self-inflicted or has resulted from barbering by a cage mate.

There is no specific treatment other than removal of an offending animal for either a generalized diffuse alopecia or hair loss from barbering; however, providing good quality hay may be of some benefit, particularly in the case of barbering. Measures to reduce stress levels should also be considered.

Circumanal Sebaceous Accumulations

Excessive accumulations of sebaceous secretions occur in the folds of the circumanal and genital region in adult male guinea pigs. These folds must be cleansed periodically to preclude infection and unpleasant odors (Wagner 1976). At times the sebaceous secretions form a plug that accumulates in the folds between the two halves of the scrotum. It can be removed after softening with soap and water (Williams 1976).

Preputial Infection and Vaginitis

Male guinea pigs occasionally develop preputial infections caused by lodging of foreign material in the preputial folds. Breeding males on bedding may be affected when pieces of bedding adhere to the moist prepuce following copulation and are drawn into the preputial fornix. Treatment primarily involves removing the particle and cleansing the area.

Vaginitis in female guinea pigs is usually caused by entrapment of wood chips or other bedding in the vagina, causing a foreign body reaction. The problem is corrected by washing the area carefully and swabbing away the chips. It may be desirable to place the animal on a different type of bedding until the area has healed.

Water Deprivation

Sometimes animals die of water deprivation even when ample water seems to be available (Wagner 1976). This may occur when (1) water is provided by a device with which the animal is not familiar or does not know how to operate, (2) water devices are placed too high or are otherwise inaccessible, particularly for small weanlings, (3) water is unpotable because of impurities or odors in the container or the water itself, (4) automatic watering devices or sipper tubes become inoperable from plugging with foreign objects or air locks, and (5) territorialism on the part of dominant individuals prevents less agressive animals from drinking.

CHAPTER 6

RABBITS

CHARACTERISTICS

Laboratory rabbits belong to the order Lagomorpha and are referred to collectively as lagomorphs. The scientific name of the domestic rabbit is *Oryctolagus cuniculus*. Hares (*Lepus*) and cottontails (*Sylvilagus*) are in different genera.

Domestic rabbits resemble rodents in many respects. The principal anatomic feature differentiating rodents from rabbits is that rabbits have two pairs of upper incisor teeth, while rodents have only one pair (Flatt 1977a). The additional pair in rabbits is reduced in size and located directly behind the front pair.

Breeds

At the present time the American Rabbit Breeders Association recognizes 28 different breeds and 77 varieties of rabbits (Harkness and Wagner 1977). The more popular breeds are described below:

1. New Zealand White is the most popular breed of rabbit for research purposes and meat production.
2. American Dutch is second in importance as a laboratory breed. It is smaller than the New Zealand breed and therefore can be housed in smaller cages.
3. California is another large breed that is differentiated from the New Zealand White by its dark ears, nose, and feet. It is used for meat production.
4. Other breeds not used in significant numbers in the laboratory but kept mainly for pets and show include the American Chinchilla, Satin, Rex, Silver Martin, American Checkered Giant, Polish, and Lop.

Uses

Rabbits are growing in popularity as pets and for hobby breeding. They are clean, attractive, relatively easy to handle, and can grow to enjoy the attention given them as pets. They seldom bite but can inflict deep scratches if not properly held.

Although domestic rabbit meat cannot be produced as economically as poultry, 25-30 million lbs/yr are consumed in the United States (Flatt 1977a), and the popularity of rabbits as a source of meat is expected to increase.

Rabbits are used in substantial numbers for research and drug testing. Their size, ease of handling, and large ear veins make them very suitable for many studies. The rabbit is a particularly popular laboratory animal for the immunologist because they are good antibody producers and their blood is relatively easy to collect.

BIOLOGY

Normal physiologic data is given in App. 2. Among the important physiologic facts are (1) life span, 5-13 yr; (2) breeding age, 6-9 mo; (3) gestation period, 31 days (range 28-35 days); (4) weaning age, 6-8 wks; and (5) average normal rectal temperature, 102.5°F.

Anatomic Features

The presence of an extra pair of upper incisors has already been mentioned. The purpose of these short cylindrical teeth is not clear.

The sacculus rotundus is an enlargement of the terminal end of the ileum where it joins the cecum, and contains lymphoid tissue, giving it a pale appearance. It is the counterpart of the bursa of Fabricius in chickens.

The genital tract of a doe, like that of most domestic animals, is bicornuate but differs in that there is also a double cervix with the two horns of the uterus opening into the vagina through separate cervices. The uterine horns are curled and lie in the caudal abdomen dorsal to the urinary bladder (Sedgwick 1982).

The rabbit skeleton is only about 7% of its body weight compared to a cat skeleton, which is 13% of its body weight (Harkness and Wagner 1977). For this reason and because of heavy muscles in the back and rear legs, fractures are common, particularly of the lumbar spine.

Rabbit neutrophils have intracytoplasmic eosinophilic granules that cause them to resemble eosinophils; they are called "pseudoeosinophils" or "heterophils." True eosinophils have larger, darker granules than heterophils.

Lateral to the external genitalia are the paired, hairless inguinal spaces, usually containing whitish to brownish secretions from the inguinal glands. Someone unfamiliar with rabbit anatomy could conceivably mistake an inguinal space for the anus.

Physiology

Rabbits pass two types of feces: the firm, dry daytime feces and the soft, moist nighttime fecal pellet. The night feces are covered with mucus and composed mainly of secretion from the cecum. They are taken directly from the anus and swallowed intact by the rabbit. The soft pellets contain twice the protein and half the fiber of the hard fecal pellets. The process improves the utilization of nitrogen, provides an abundance of certain B vitamins, and conserves water.

Rabbit urine may range in color from cloudy yellow to red brown; normal urine thus may resemble a purulent discharge. The carbonate and phosphate crystals cause a scale on cages, which is best removed by soaking or rinsing in an acid solution.

Atropine esterase, which hydrolyzes atropine, is present in the serum of about one-third of the domestic rabbit population. As a result of the presence of atropine esterase, these animals are refractory to administration of atropine.

Reproduction

Differentiating males from females can be accomplished readily in adults by gently pressing the skin back from the genital opening. The female has a short slitlike opening, and pressing the skin back exposes the mucosal surface of the vulva. In the male, this procedure will cause the penis to be everted. In the mature male, inguinal pouches (the scrotum) can be located lateral and anterior to the penis. In the newborn, when pressure is applied against the genital orifice, the penis will evert equally all the way around while the vulva protrudes only laterally and ventrally; the posterior end which does not evert is closely attached near the anus (Williams 1976).

Rabbits do not have a definite estrus cycle but have short periods (1-2 days) about every 2 wk in which they are not receptive to the male. On occasion, a doe will refuse to mate with one buck but will readily accept another. She also may accept a buck once but refuse him a second time (Hagen 1974).

In the wild, courtship chasing between adults is an early form of sexual activity. Caged rabbits are denied this opportunity and their courtship antics are restricted to tail flagging and enurination (Hagen 1974). Tail flagging is a common form of behavior. The buck elevates his hindquarters, walks stiff-legged, and lays his tail flat across his back. This maneuver supplies a visual stimulus to the doe as well as an olfactory stimulus from the inguinal glands. Enurination is the process of emitting a jet of urine in a display of sexual aggressiveness. The buck may turn his hindquarters toward a doe and eject a small amount of urine; this is followed by some form of circling about the cage. The urine may also be directed at another male in an adjacent cage.

When breeding rabbits, the female should ordinarily be taken to the male's cage. Copulation will take place soon after introduction of the male if the female is receptive. After ejaculation, the male will usually fall off either to the side or backward. Slow motion photography has revealed that this loss of balance results because both feet are off the ground simultaneously at the time of ejaculation (Hagen 1974). Approximately 10 hr after mating, the doe will ovulate as a result of the stimulation of mating (induced ovulation). Mounting by other does may also stimulate ovulation and result in pseudopregnancy. Ovulation can be induced by administration of human chorionic gonadotropins (Rx: F.3.e) or other luteinizing hormones if a producer wishes to employ artificial insemination.

Parturition is called "kindling." Litters usually consist of 6-7 rabbits. The young normally nurse only once a day. Their eyes open at 10 days, they begin to eat solid food at about 3 wk of age, and they may be weaned at 6-8 wk.

Orphaned rabbits can be fed orphaned puppy formula with a syringe, doll bottle, or gastric intubation. Milk should be offered 3 times a day, giving up to 5 ml/day the first week, 15 ml/day the second week, and 25 ml/day the third week (Harkness and Wagner 1977). Newborn rabbits do not require colostrum because all passive immunity is acquired through the placenta (Williams 1976).

HUSBANDRY

Housing

Most commercial producers house rabbits in wire mesh hanging cages.

Nest boxes are placed in these cages near the end of gestation for birth of the young (kindling). In the research laboratory rabbits are usually housed in stainless steel cages with slotted sides, wire grid fronts and mesh or grid floors with excreta trays beneath. Automatic water systems are great laborsavers, both for production colonies and in the research laboratory.

Environmental Requirements

For indoor housing of rabbits, heat is not required. However, the temperature is usually kept in the range of 65-75°F; if the ambient temperature exceeds 85°F, auxiliary ventilation is required. Ventilation must be adequate to maintain health and minimize draft and odors. Animal rooms should have 10-15 air changes/hr, depending on the density of the animals. The desired relative humidity is around 50%. Sufficient light is required to permit cleaning and inspection. Light is usually provided for 12-14 hr/day.

TECHNIQUES

Restraint and Handling

Rabbits should be handled gently but firmly. They are prone to kick their hind legs and can cause deep scratches. A rabbit should be picked up by obtaining a firm grip on the loose skin over the scruff of the neck with one hand while using the other to support the animal's hindquarters and control back leg movement. If the hind legs are not supported, the rabbit may break its back in struggling. The ears should not be used in picking up a rabbit.

If pet rabbits are to be handled by small children, a declawing operation, following a technique similar to that employed to declaw cats, may be advisable (Williams 1976).

To carry a rabbit, it should be placed on the forearm with its head concealed in the bend of the elbow.

Rabbits feel insecure and will slip and slide on stainless steel examining tables. Placing the animal on a bath towel or wrapping it will make the rabbit calmer and easier to handle. In examining the underside of a rabbit, gently stroking downward on the abdomen will have a calming affect (Williams 1979).

Restraining boxes of many designs are available. They primarily serve to control the body of the rabbit while the head or ears are being manipulated.

Oral Medication

Palatable drugs may be administered to rabbits by incorporating them in the food or water. Small volumes of liquid materials can be administered by placing the tip of a syringe in the corner of the mouth and slowly injecting the liquid (Bivin and Timmons 1974). Oral administration of liquids having an unpleasant taste may be accomplished using a stomach tube passed through a nostril or the mouth. If passed through the mouth, some means of preventing damage to the tube by the rabbit's teeth is required. A mouth gag can be fashioned from a wooden dowel or tongue depressor having a hole of sufficient diameter for passage of the tube. Another means of gastric intubation is the use of a 13-gauge, 16-in. stainless steel feeding needle (Feldman 1977).

Blood Collection and Intravenous Injections

The marginal ear vein, which courses along the posterior margin of the ear, is a convenient site for blood collection and intravenous injections. The auricular artery may also be used for blood collection.

Cardiac punctures can be used to collect larger quantities of blood. To collect blood by heart puncture, the animal should be anesthetized or sedated.

Anesthesia

See section F.4 of App. 1 for anesthetic agents and dosages.

Caution should be exercised in anesthetizing rabbits, particularly when using barbiturates, because of the narrow margin between surgical anesthesia and death. The depth of anesthesia is best gauged by the rate and depth of respiration and degree of jaw tension; the pedal reflex, corneal reflex, and pupillary size are unreliable indicators.

BACTERIAL DISEASES

Pasteurellosis

Pasteurellosis is the single most common and troublesome disease of domestic rabbits. It is caused by *Pasteurella multocida*. Clinical signs may range from peracute septicemic death to chronic abscessation or rhinitis.

Many rabbits harbor the organism in the respiratory tract without showing clinical signs. Following stress, a variety of syndromes may develop in infected rabbits: rhinitis, conjunctivitis, pneumonia, otitis media and interna, genital infections, abscesses, and septicemia.

Snuffles (rhinitis) is the upper respiratory form of pasteurellosis, characterized by sneezing and the presence of a mucopurulent nasal exudate. Rabbits frequently will use their forelimbs to wipe their noses as the exudate begins to accumulate, and exudate will then be seen on the inner aspect of the forelegs. Animals may live for many months with snuffles, or the disease may progress to one of the other clinical forms.

A subacute to chronic conjunctivitis or epiphora may be a clinical manifestation of *P. multocida* infection, with resultant loss of fur around the medial canthus of the eye.

Snuffles may progress to the pulmonary form of pasteurellosis and appear as acute pneumonia with consolidation of the lungs. Cyanosis is often a prominent feature of pneumonia in rabbits. At times, rabbits will die of acute pneumonia without observable clinical signs.

The organisms may spread from the nasal passage to the middle and inner ear. When the infection reaches the inner ear, there will be balance problems and torticollis, commonly called "head tilt" or "wry neck." The head tilt may be so severe that the head is nearly upside down. Most cases of otitis interna are caused by *P. multocida* infections.

Genital infections in rabbits include pyometra in the doe and orchitis in the buck. With pyometra the exudate is yellow-white and has a thick, creamy consistency. Venereal transmission occurs during breeding.

Large subcutaneous abscesses may be seen with *P. multocida* infections. The abscess contents tend to be very thick and in some instances is more readily removed by scooping than by aspiration.

The organism is usually sensitive to a number of antibiotics; but they rarely provide a complete bacteriologic cure. The organisms are harbored in the nasal passages and, although remission following antibiotic therapy is common, infection is usually reestablished after discontinuation of treatment (Jaslow et al. 1981). Antibiotics often used in treating pasteurellosis include chlortetracycline (Rx: F.1.e), oxytetracycline (Rx: F.1.k), penicillin (Rx: F.1.n), ampicillin (Rx: F.1.a), and chloramphenicol (Rx: F.1.c; F.1.d). A degree of caution should be exercised in using antibiotics for prolonged periods because of the possibility of treated animals developing a fatal diarrhea (Rehg and Lu 1981).

Complete elimination of P. multocida infections in commercial rabbitries is not likely to be achieved. Breeders generally direct their efforts toward avoiding spread of infection and minimizing the incidence of clinical disease. This is mainly a matter of (1) quarantine of incoming animals; (2) elimination of environmental stressors, giving particular attention to adequate ventilation; (3) isolation or culling of affected animals; and (4) providing medicated feeds, the use of which is indicated at times but should not be used to compensate for poor husbandry practices.

Cesarean derivation of breeding stock and maintenance of animals in isolation has proved a successful means of eliminating pasteurellosis but is expensive and probably practical only for research colonies. Older bacterins are of little value in preventing pasteurellosis, but new vaccines (including a streptomycin-dependent live P. multocida vaccine) show promise (Chengappa et al. 1980). None are presently available commercially. Another means of controlling pasteurellosis which is currently under study, is the development of P. multocida resistant strains. Oregon State University has developed a strain of rabbits with a high degree of natural resistance to pasteurellosis (Pasteurella-resistant rabbits 1981). This may prove a feasible method of disease control on a commercial scale.

Tyzzer's Disease

Bacillus piliformis causes an acute hemorrhagic typhlocolitis in rabbits. Stresses such as overcrowding, shipping, poor ventilation, and improper nutrition are predisposing factors. The disease is most common in rabbits 7-12 wk of age. Morbidity and mortality are usually very high, and a profuse diarrhea is characteristic. At necropsy, focal necrosis of the liver and intestinal mucosa is seen. Although Tyzzer's disease is not recognized as a common health problem in rabbits, it should be considered in the differential diagnosis of acute diarrheal disease.

Oxytetracycline (Rx: F.1.k) is suggested for treatment; however, the prognosis for animals showing clinical signs of Tyzzer's disease is very unfavorable. Institution of sound husbandry practices and elimination of environmental stress factors are crucial in controlling an outbreak in a rabbit colony.

Salmonellosis

Salmonella spp. infections are a relatively uncommon cause of enteric disease in rabbits. Clinical signs, other than diarrhea that may be evident with salmonellosis, are abortion and septicemia with rapid death (Flatt 1974).

Although nitrofurazone (Rx: F.1.j) and various other antibiotics may be effective in eliminating clinical signs of salmonellosis (USDA 1976), treatment of affected animals is not usually advisable because of the possibility that survivors may be inapparent carriers.

Venereal Spirochetosis

Venereal spirochetosis (also known as rabbit syphilis, vent disease, and treponematosis) is caused by Treponema cuniculi. The organism is serologically and morphologically similar to T. pallidum, which causes syphilis in humans; however, T. cuniculi is nonpathogenic for humans. Clinical disease is not commonly observed, although many rabbits are serologically positive. It is characterized by the presence of raised, crusted occasionally hemorrhagic, ulcerative foci on the external genitalia, perineal region, and face, particularly the nose. The disease may be confused clinically with hutch burn. At times the lesions may resemble those caused by ear mites and sarcoptic mange. Treponematosis can be differentiated from other cutaneous diseases by dark field examination of scrapings from the lesions (Cunliffe-Beamer and Fox 1981a). The disease is transmitted by direct contact, usually venereally but occasionally by extragenital routes. Three injections of benzathine penicillin G with procaine penicillin G (Rx: F.1.1) at 7-day intervals have been found effective in eliminating the infection. Affected rabbits should be isolated during the acute disease (Cunliffe-Beamer and Fox 1981b).

Mastitis

Mastitis occurs sporadically in lactating does and occasionally during pseudopregnancy. Mastitis is sometimes called "blue breast" because the skin over the mammary gland changes from pink to red then to bluish purple. *Staphylococcus aureus* is most commonly incriminated as the cause (Flatt et al. 1974). The causative organism may be introduced by means of splinters from nest boxes, trauma by the teeth of nursing young, or unsanitary housing conditions.

Treatment involves isolating the affected doe and treating her with penicillin (Rx: F.1.n) for 3-5 days. The young should be removed but not foster nursed on another doe because of the probability of spreading the disease to a healthy animal.

Miscellaneous Bacterial Infections

Necrobacillosis or Schmorl's disease (*Fusobacterium necrophorum*) is characterized by ulceration of the skin and subcutaneous swelling about the face, neck, and oral cavity (Flatt 1974). The disease incidence does not seem to be high even though *F. necrophorum* is commonly present in the digestive tract of rabbits. The infection is transmissible to humans. The recommended treatment for affected rabbits includes debridement, drainage of abscesses, systemic antibiotics such as penicillin (Rx: F.1.n) or tetracycline (Rx: F.1.r), and improved sanitation.

Tularemia (*Francisella tularensis*) usually causes sudden death of affected animals. Typical lesions at necropsy are small foci of necrosis in the spleen and liver. The disease is rare in domestic rabbits because of lack of exposure to vectors.

Listeriosis (*Listeria monocytogenes*) usually causes abortions or nonspecific signs and death. The presence of a blood-tinged vaginal discharge following abortion suggests the possibility of listeriosis. Occasionally central nervous system signs are seen. However, it is a rare disease in rabbits. Antibiotics of the tetracycline group and penicillin have been used in treating listeriosis (USDA 1976).

Pseudomonas (*Pseudomonas aeruginosa*) may produce skin infections with blue-green discoloration and occasionally involvement of other organs; but this is not a common health problem in rabbits. Infections are treated by topical application of 3% hydrogen peroxide and chlorination of drinking water (Rx: B.3.c).

Pseudotuberculosis (*Yersinia pseudotuberculosis*) typically produces caseous nodules in various organs. The disease is not commonly seen in domestic rabbits in the United States (Flatt 1974). The organism can infect humans. Treatment of pseudotuberculosis in rabbits is not usually successful.

Staphylococcal infections (*S. aureus*) may be seen as a septicemia, a dermatitis, or in various other forms. Staphylococcal infections often produce multiple abscesses in nursing bunnies maintained in unsanitary conditions (Russell 1981). Chloramphenicol (Rx: F.1.c; F.1.d), gentamicin (Rx: F.1.h), or tetracycline (Rx: F.1.r) in conjunction with topical treatment is sometimes effective; however, antibiotic treatment of staphylococcal infections is frequently discouraging (Russell 1981).

ENTERIC DISEASES OF UNCERTAIN ETIOLOGY

As a group, enteric diseases are second only to pasteurellosis as a health problem in domestic rabbits. The enteric diseases are probably the least understood of the common diseases encountered. In some cases diarrhea is caused by a specific, well-defined agent; but the cause of enteric disease in rabbits is frequently obscure.

Specific enteric diseases include coccidiosis, Tyzzer's disease, and salmonellosis. Those of uncertain etiologies include colibacillosis, enterotoxemia, and mucoid enteropathy.

Colibacillosis

Colibacillosis might appropriately be classified as a specific enteric disease; however, the role of the *Escherichia coli* organism is not completely understood. It is known that *E. coli* is either absent or present in low numbers in the gut of normal rabbits, but that in some cases of severe diarrhea, the organisms are isolated in large numbers (Williams 1976). It is generally thought, however, that *E. coli* is a secondary agent rather than the primary cause of disease.

Treatment is largely symptomatic. Systemic and parenteral antibiotics, intestinal protectants, fluids and electrolytes, and other supportive measures may be beneficial. Alteration of the diet (reducing the amount of concentrates fed to no more that 2-3 oz/day and providing added roughage such as hay) is often more effective than antibiotics in reducing mortality.

Enterotoxemia

As with colibacillosis, some consider enterotoxemia as a specific enteric disease and there is supportive evidence for this. *Clostridium perfringens*, type E toxin, has been recovered from intestinal contents of rabbits dying of acute enteritis. A hemorrhagic and edematous cecum is typically seen in these cases (Patton et al. 1978). Possibly a virus is the triggering agent for colibacillosis or enterotoxemia. It has been speculated that a virus damages the epithelial cells of the intestine, which gives rise to a disturbance in the cecal water metabolism. This, along with a depression in antibacterial resistance, favors the increased growth of toxin producing bacteria such as *E. coli* and *C. perfringens*. Thus two organisms, a virus and a bacteria, are required (Patton 1981).

Mucoid Enteropathy

Mucoid enteropathy is a frequent disease problem in young rabbits. Whether it is a distinctive disease with a specific etiology is not clear; it may be merely a syndrome caused by a number of different agents. Two characteristic features of this disease are the presence of clear gelatinous material in the colon and the relatively noninflammatory nature of the lesion in the intestinal mucosa. The reaction is primarily an increased production of goblet cells; thus it is properly classified as an enteropathy rather than an enteritis.

The disease most commonly affects rabbits from 3-10 wk of age. Affected animals usually exhibit abdominal distention, dehydration, subnormal temperature, and staining of perineal fur with liquid feces. A splashing noise may be heard when an affected rabbit is picked up.

Suspected causes of mucoid enteropathy include (1) transition from milk to a solid diet (amylase deficiency), (2) *E. coli*, (3) *C. perfringes* and other enterotoxins, (4) rotavirus, (5) genetic inborn errors of metabolism, (6) stress and (7) combination of two or more of the preceding.

Measures recommended for the prevention of mucoid enteropathy follow:

1. Practice good sanitation.
2. Eliminate stressors where possible.
3. Increase fiber content of the diet by reducing concentrates and feeding hay or straw, although excessively high fiber diets (i.e., greater than 20% fiber) should be avoided because they reduce the growth rate of young rabbits and may cause digestive disturbances (Patton and Cheeke 1981). Coarse fibrous materials may be more effective than finely ground fiber in preventing mucoid enteropathy and other nonspecific enteric disorders.
4. Vaccination is of questionable value, although there have been reports of beneficial results from administering Scourvac II to rabbits at 1 wk of age, giving 0.10 ml orally of the double strength vaccine (Willis and Jensen 1979); however, the validity of these reports is uncertain.
5. Culling does with affected litters has been suggested, although evidence of a genetic predisposition has not been clearly established.

Treatment is usually not very rewarding once symptoms have developed. Medication used in prevention and treatment include chlortetracycline (Rx: F.1.e) with continuous feeding beginning at 2 wk of age and continuing to 8 wk of age (Flatt et al. 1974) and nitrofurazone (Rx: F.1.j) and dimetridazole (Rx: F.1.f) for 1 wk before and after weaning. Fluid and electrolyte therapy is indicated if justified by the value of the animal. Appropriate measures should be taken to eliminate any complicating factors such as a concurrent coccidial infection.

VIRAL DISEASES

Myxomatosis (poxvirus)

Myxomatosis is characterized by the appearance of a conjunctivitis and gelatinous subcutaneous swellings, particularly about the face, ears, and external genitalia. In the United States the disease occurs only in the western parts of the country. The virus is usually transmitted by mosquitoes or another arthropod vector.

Shope fibromatosis (poxvirus)

The lesions of fibromatosis appear as subcutaneous nodules on various parts of the body. Natural cases are usually restricted to cottontails. This virus is antigenically related to the myxomatosis virus.

Oral papillomatosis (papovavirus)

Lesions of oral papillomatosis are seen as whitish discrete growths, usually on the underside of the tongue.

Cutaneous papillomatosis (papovavirus)

Infection with the virus causing cutaneous papillomatosis results in formation of horny warts, usually on the neck, shoulder or abdomen. Lesions are seen primarily in cottontails.

Cardiomyopathy

A cardiomyopathy caused by a coronavirus has been reported. The hearts of affected animals exhibit myocardial necrosis and degeneration with little inflammatory response (Small et al. 1979).

PARASITIC DISEASES

Ear Mites

Psoroptes cuniculi is the cause of ear canker (otitis externa) in rabbits. This condition is very common in rabbits from conventional colonies. Ear mite infection is characterized by the presence of dry, brown crusty material on the inner surface of the ear. In advanced cases the crusts are readily apparent without the aid of an otoscope.

Treatment involves generous application of mineral oil with or without miticides. A mixture of 1 part Canex (a rotenone preparation) and 3 parts mineral oil has been commonly used in the past; however, Canex is apparently no longer available. In severe cases the ear canal should be gently cleansed prior to medication with a miticide. Treatment must be repeated 3 or 4 times weekly to kill the newly hatched mites.

Mange Mites

Although, rabbits are susceptible to *Notoedres cati* and *Sarcoptes scabiei*, these mites do not commonly cause infection.

Fur Mites

Cheyletiella parasitovorax is the fur mite or rabbits. This parasite causes thinning of the fur and scaly lesions, having the appearance of dandruff, down the back of an affected animal. Because it does not burrow, the mite is easily killed with cat flea powder. Infection resulting in dermatitis has been reported in humans (Flatt 1977b).

Cuterebra

Cuterebra larvae appear as large lumps with perforated breathing holes in the subcutaneous tissue. They grow up to 1 in. long and are similar in appearance to ox warbles. Treatment consists of incising the skin and removing the larva.

Roundworms

The rabbit pinworm, *Passaluris ambiguus*, is a whitish hairlike worm that can be seen in the rabbit's cecal contents and is voided in the feces. Pinworms are not considered very pathogenic to rabbits and are not infective to humans. They can be treated with piperazine adipate (Rx: F.2.e) given for 2 days in the feed or water or fenbendazole (Rx: F.2.b) in the feed for 5 days.

Obeliscoides cuniculi and *Trichostrongylus calcaratus* are roundworms that inhabit the digestive tract of rabbits. Infections are rarely encountered in commercial operations. Control can be achieved by employment of good sanitation practices (USDA 1976).

Tapeworms

The rabbit tapeworm, *Cittotaenia ctenoides*, seldom causes clinical problems and can be controlled by proper sanitation (USDA 1976). Niclosamide (Rx: F.2.c) is effective against the rabbit tapeworm (Williams 1979).

Larval forms of _Taenia piliformis_ may be found in the abdominal cavity or liver of rabbits ingesting food or water contaminated by dog or cat feces (Brooks 1979).

Protozoa

Encephalitozoonosis is a disease caused by the protozoan organism _Encephalitozoan cuniculi_, formerly called _Nosema cuniculi_. This agent commonly infects domestic rabbits and is occasionally found in other species. It is primarily important as a complicating factor in interpretation of experimental data. The organisms grow in the epithelium of the kidney tubule and eventually cause fibrosis and pitting of the cortex (Flatt 1977b). Lesions in the brain require microscopic examination for detection and seldom cause clinical signs.

Coccidiosis

Coccidiosis is common in conventional rabbit colonies. Rabbits are susceptible to the hepatic type caused by _Eimeria stiedae_ and the intestinal type caused by several species of _Eimeria_, including _E. magna_, _E. perforans_, _E. media_, and _E. irresidua_. The intestinal type is by far the most common.

Adult rabbits usually show no clinical signs from infection with _E. stiedae_; but heavy infections in young animals may cause weight loss, diarrhea, and a potbellied appearance. At necropsy the liver is enlarged and contains irregularly shaped, slightly raised yellow-white foci (Harkness and Wagner 1977). Microscopically, bile duct hyperplasia and inflammation can be seen.

In mild cases of intestinal coccidiosis, few if any clinical signs are evident. Weight gains may be poor, and the fecal material may be formed but softer than normal and tend to stick to the wires of the cage floor. When present, diarrhea may range from an intermittent to a profuse watery form with traces of blood. Deaths that occur are usually in younger animals.

The life cycle is direct, as in other species. Transmission occurs through the ingestion of sporulated infective oocysts. Sporulation can occur in as little as 2 days if the ambient temperature and humidity are optimal. Reingestion of the soft nighttime fecal pellets does not allow time for sporulation; therefore, infection by this route is unlikely (Harkness and Wagner 1977). With both intestinal and hepatic coccidiosis, oocysts appear in the feces except in animals that die very soon after onset of illness. A yeast, _Saccharomycopsis guttulata_ is commonly found in rabbit feces and should not be incorrectly identified as a coccidial oocyte (Williams 1976).

Prevention and control of coccidiosis is achieved by (1) strict cleaning and disinfectant procedures (a 10% household ammonia solution is an effective disinfectant) (Brooks 1979); (2) use of wire hanging cages, J type feeders and water bottles or automatic watering devices; (3) medicated feed or water; and (4) culling of infected animals, which is indicated under some circumstances.

There is no effective treatment for elimination of _E. stediae_ from the liver, but medication can be helpful in preventing the initial infection. Among the drugs used for treating or preventing coccidiosis are sulfamethazine (Rx: F.1.p), sulfadimethoxide (Rx: F.1.o), sulfaquinoxaline (Rx: F.1.q), amprolium (Rx: F.2.a), and furazolidone (Rx: F.1.g).

MYCOTIC DISEASES

Dermatophytosis

Ringworm in rabbits is most frequently caused by *Trichophyton mentagrophytes*. Since *T. mentagrophytes* does not fluoresce under ultraviolet light, microscopic examination or culturing of hair or skin scrapings is usually required to establish a diagnosis. Lesions are pruritic, crusty, and hairless and in most cases first appear on the head or ears. Ringworm is not often encountered in domestic rabbits except in animals housed under poor husbandry conditions (Flatt et al. 1974).

Lesions may be treated with topical antifungal creams applied twice daily (often for 4 wk or longer) or by administration of griseofulvin orally (Rx: F.1.i).

Systemic Mycoses

Systemic fungal infections have been infrequently reported in rabbits (Russell et al. 1981).

MISCELLANEOUS CONDITIONS

Malocclusion

Tooth overgrowth results when open-rooted teeth do not properly occlude and therefore are not worn away. The condition has a genetic basis and is due to a shortening of the upper jaw. This causes the lower incisors to grow anterior instead of posterior to the upper teeth. Overgrown incisors may be treated by trimming them with toenail trimmers, bone cutters, or a motorized tool (e.g., Dremel). The rough edges may be smoothed with a nail file. Repeated clipping of the lower teeth will never cure the condition, and culling of an affected animal and its offspring is the only succesful means of eradication in a breeding group.

Fracture or Luxation of the Lumbar Spine

A sudden onset of posterior paralysis in a rabbit strongly suggests a fracture or luxation of the lumbar spine. This commonly occurs in rabbits that are dropped or allowed to thrash during attempted restraint. Usually it is due to failure to support the hindquarters.

The prognosis after back injury depends on the location and severity of the cord lesion but is usually unfavorable. Occasionally an animal will recover with cage rest, but in most cases posterior paralysis with urinary incontinence persists and euthanasia is required.

Moist Dermatitis

Two forms of moist dermatitis that occur in rabbits are "sore dewlap" and "hutch burn." Various bacteria may be involved, but the underlying cause of these conditions is constant wetting of fur.

The usual conditions that lead to sore dewlap are drooling from malocclusion or drinking from open pans or crocks (Williams 1979). Treatment consists of clipping the fur from the affected area and applying hydrogen peroxide or a topical ointment.

Hutch burn is a superficial inflammatory condition of the anogenital area caused by prolonged contact of the skin with urine or soiling by diarrhea (Williams 1979). To treat, eliminate the underlying cause (which is primarily a matter of correcting husbandry practices); cleanse the lesion; and apply topical medication such as an antibiotic ointment.

Hair Balls (Gastric Trichobezoars)

Gastric hair balls should be suspected in rabbits that suddenly stop eating and drinking and pass no fecal material but otherwise appear alert and in good health. The presence of a hair ball can usually be detected by palpation; however, in some cases, a radiograph (with or without barium) may be necessary to confirm the diagnosis. Hair balls are in most cases the result of excessive self-grooming, often attributed to boredom; however, deficiencies of copper, magnesium, certain amino acids, and fiber have been suggested as contributing causes. The incidence may be high in recently purchased animals as a result of molting presumably due to a change in diet and room temperature.

Providing roughage such as alfalfa hay, apples, or cabbage is beneficial in prevention of hair balls and may on some occasions assist in the passage of masses of hair. High fiber (up to 20%) pellets rather than other forms of roughage may be used to provide bulk.

Mineral oil (10-15 ml) may be administered by means of a stomach tube but is seldom effective in elimination of large hair balls.

Removal of a hair ball surgically may be indicated with a valuable animal. A relatively high degree of success following surgical intervention can be anticipated if excessive delay does not occur prior to surgery; proper provisions are made for maintaining body temperature during and following surgery; and appropriate steps are taken to prevent or treat ketosis, such as administration of 50% dextrose (Rx: F.3.d). Death following blockage of the stomach by a hair ball is usually attributable to ketosis.

Uterine Adenocarcinoma

The most common neoplasm of domestic rabbits is uterine adenocarcinoma (Weisbroth 1974). The incidence of uterine adenocarcinoma is very high in does 5 yr of age and older. A doe's reproductive performance generally declines several months prior to the time the tumor can be detected clinically (Harkness and Wagner 1977). Metastasis to the lung and other organs occasionally occurs (Timm et al. 1979). Because of frequency of uterine neoplasia in mature does, an ovariohysterectomy should be considered for pets not used for breeding. The surgical procedure is performed in a manner similar to ovariohysterectomy in a cat; however, the abdomonal wall is comparatively thin in a rabbit and retraction of the cecum and urinary bladder may be necessary to expose the uterine horns (Sedgwick 1982).

Heat Stroke

Rabbits are very susceptible to overheating, and heavy losses may result from heat stroke. Young rabbits in nest boxes are particularly prone. Rabbits housed out doors should be provided shade and those indoors should have good ventilation.

Buphthalmia

Buphthalmia is a form of glaucoma that is one of the more common inherited diseases of domestic rabbits (Lindsey and Fox 1974). With this disease there is an increase in the size of the anterior chamber, resulting in corneal opacity and increased prominence of the eyeball. Treatment of affected individuals would not ordinarily seem feasible.

Splay Leg

An abnormality in which a rabbit is unable to adduce one or more limbs is called splay leg (Lindsey and Fox 1974). The most common cause is subluxation of the hip. Affected animals sit with their legs sticking out sideways. Splay leg is usually due to a recessive inherited trait. There is no effective treatment and prevention is accomplished by culling animals carrying this trait.

Muscular Dystrophy

Vitamin E deficiencies can result in nutritional muscular dystrophy. Clinical signs are neonatal mortality, infertility, keratitis, and muscular weakness in growing rabbits (Russell 1981). Commercial diets usually provide adequate amounts of vitamin E.

Ulcerative Pododermatitis

Ulcerative pododermatitis is also called "sore hock," but it actually involves the ventral metatarsal region rather than the hock. It usually occurs in heavy rabbits maintained on wire mesh floors. The condition may also occur if rabbits are nervous and stamp their feet or if solid floors become urine soaked.

The lesion consists of a circumscribed ulcerated area in the skin which is covered by a dry crusty scab. Abscesses may form under the scab. *Staphylococcus aureus* is a frequent cause of these abscesses (Flatt et al. 1974). Affected individuals may lose weight and sit in a humped-up position or shift weight on their hind feet.

Treatment consists of providing soft, clean bedding; clean, dry, solid-bottom cages; or a piece of wood in the cage for the rabbit to sit on. Lesions may be treated by application of a topical ointment such as zinc oxide. A bandage affords protection against further trauma. If abscesses are present, systemic antibiotics such as penicillin (Rx: F.1.n) are indicated.

Ketosis (Pregnancy Toxemia)

Ketosis occasionally occurs in rabbits and in most cases is seen in obese does a few days prior to parturition. It is analogous to ketosis in guinea pigs and sheep in terms of etiology, treatment, and prevention (see discussion for ketosis in guinea pigs).

CHAPTER 7

FERRETS

CHARACTERISTICS

The ferret (Mustela putorius furo) is a carnivore related to the skunk, weasel, and mink. It was domesticated from the wild European polecat. There are two varieties of domestic ferret; the pale yellow-buff wild type or fitch with a black mask, limbs, and tail and the albino, which is white with pink eyes when young but becomes more yellow as it matures because of sebaceous secretions from its skin. The domestic ferret should not be confused with the native North American black-footed ferret (Mustela nigripes).

Uses

According to the most recent figures available, approximately 12,000 ferrets are sold each year in the United States - about half to the pet trade and half to research laboratories. There was a fivefold increase in the sale of ferrets in the United States during the five years preceding the survey. Their popularity as pets has continued to increase. Ferrets tend to have a friendly disposition and make suitable though not particularly exciting pets. Like cats, they spend much time sleeping. An objectional feature of ferrets is the musky odor from the anal scent glands, which is emitted when an animal is excited or angry. These can be removed surgically, but even then a slight musky odor from skin secretions will persist (Ryland and Gorham 1978). Some states have laws that prohibit or regulate the keeping of ferrets. If a ferret should escape and gain access to a poultry house, a heavy loss of birds can be anticipated. Ferrets will kill for sport and eat very little of their prey.

Although not used in large numbers for research, ferrets are valuable in a number of areas, including studies of the physiology of reproduction, virus-induced neoplasms, bacterial infections, and viral diseases of humans and other animals. They have been particularly useful for studies of canine distemper, vesicular stomatitis, and human influenza. They are currently used as a model system for studies of drugs effective in providing symptomatic relief of the common cold (Williams 1976).

BIOLOGY

Anatomic Feature

Emphysematous pulmonary foci (small, pale yellow, slightly elevated spots) may be seen on the surface of the lungs at necropsy. These lesions are foci of subpleural emphysema with accumulations of macrophages in the alveoli (Hammond and Chesterman 1976) and are of no known clinical significance.

Physiology

Normal physiologic values are listed in App. 2. Of particular importance to the clinical veterinarian are the following considerations.

The normal rectal temperature is in the range 101-102.5°F but excitement may raise this to 104°F.

Ferrets normally live for 5-6 yr, although life spans of 8-9 yr are common (Ryland and Gorham 1978).

Large seasonal fluctations in weight are due to the accumulation of subcutaneous fat in the autumn and its subsequent loss in the spring and summer.

Hematocrit values, hemoglobin levels, erythrocyte counts, and reticulocyte counts tend to be somewhat higher in ferrets than in other species of laboratory animals, and the average values for males are slightly higher than for females in all except reticulocyte counts (Thornton et al. 1979).

Slight to moderate proteinuria is commonly found in ferrets. The naturally dark urine of the male may present difficulty in interpretation of urine chemistry tests when colorimetric methods are used (Thornton et al. 1979).

HUSBANDRY

Housing

Ferrets tolerate low temperatures without difficulty; however, because adults do not have well-developed sweat glands, they are prone to heat exhaustion. Because of this, ferrets should be housed out of direct sunlight and provided adequate air circulation.

Ferrets seem to enjoy a den box with a small entry hole. They will habitually use one corner of the cage for droppings, and a pet ferret can be trained to use a litter box.

Nutrition

Mink wet mix or pellets are satisfactory as a diet for ferrets. They also thrive on a diet of canned or dry dog or cat food fed ad libitum. Swine pellets containing added copper should not be fed (Williams 1976). Cod liver oil, 3-5 drops a day, may be added to the diet if the coat becomes dry (Ryland and Gorham 1978). Providing free-choice salt is a common practice. Milk and bread are palatable additions to the diet; however, such a diet may cause loose, smelly feces (Williams 1976).

Reproduction

Sexing of ferrets is accomplished without difficulty since the penis is situated on the ventral abdomen. Male ferrets are called "hobs" and females, "jills."

Ferrets reach sexual maturity in the spring after their birth or at approximately 1 yr of age (Ryland and Gorham 1978). The breeding season is from March to August. As March approaches, the testicles of the males enlarge and descend into the scrotum and the vulva of the female shows a pronounced swelling. As in the rabbit, ovulation is induced. Unless the female is mated, she will remain in a state of constant estrus throughout the breeding season. A protracted period of estrus is characterized by weight loss, increased susceptibility to uterine infections, and aplastic anemia. These features probably account for a common belief that unmated females will pine away and die.

Mating is a very dramatic affair with a certain amount of rolling and jumping, the female submitting to being dragged around the cage by the scruff of the neck. Copulation last from 1-3 hr. Part of this time is spend in achieving intromission because the males are poorly coordinated. Ovulation takes place 30-40 hr after mating (Hammond and Chesterman 1976).

The duration of both pseudopregnancy and pregnancy is 40-42 days (Hammond and Chesterman 1976). Litter size ranges from 2 to 17. The young, referred to as "kits," are born hairless and blind. Their eyes and ears open at 21-37 days of age (Ryland and Bernard 1983), they are weaned at 6-8 wk, and reach their adult weight at about 4 mo (Ryland and Gorham 1978). The female will return to estrus after the young are weaned, thereby allowing production of two litters annually.

TECHNIQUES

Restraint and Handling

Most ferrets are gentle and can be handled without gloves, but sick animals or females with young should be handled with caution. The ferret may be picked up by placing a hand across the shoulders, the thumb under the chin, the forefinger around the neck, and the other fingers around the chest behind the forelimbs. Or a ferret may be picked up by grasping the loose skin at the nape of the neck with one hand while supporting the hindquarters with the other.

Blood Collection

The ferret has no readily accessible blood vessels for intravenous injection or blood withdrawal. Clipping a toenail is usually sufficient for collection of small amounts of blood; jugular venipuncture or cardiac tap in an anesthetized animal can be used for larger amounts.

Drug Administration

Intramuscular injections are given as in the dog or cat. In the fall, allowance should be made for the thick layer of subcutaneous fat that requires a longer needle to deliver an injection to muscles of the rear leg or elsewhere. Subcutaneous injections can be made in the dorsal cervical area. Oral dosing of unpalatable drugs is accomplished by using a dowel rod with a hole in it placed behind the canine teeth to serve as a mouth gag and to permit introduction of a stomach tube.

Immunization

Ferrets must be routinely protected against canine distemper by vaccination with modified live virus of chicken embryo origin, which has been found superior to formalin-inactivated vaccines (Baker et al. 1952). Live vaccines of ferret origin are not recommended. The initial dose should be administered at 6-8 wk of age if the dam has been immunized or 4-6 wk if kits are from susceptible, unvaccinated dams. The initial dose should be followed by a booster 2 wk later. Booster injections should be given every third year thereafter (Ryland and Bernard 1983). Some prefer to vaccinate at 8, 10, 12, and 16 wk of age and annually thereafter (Welch 1983). Because distemper is almost invariably fatal, a ferret should be vaccinated at the time of its first visit to a veterinary hospital unless previously immunized or exhibiting signs of the disease.

Rabies vaccine, killed only and of murine origin, can be administered annually beginning at 3 mo of age (Ryland and Gorham 1978). There is not complete agreement on the issue of vaccinating ferrets against rabies; but if one elects to immunize, a modified live rabies virus vaccine _must not be used_.

Ferrets raised commercially are usually inoculated at weaning time with type C botulism toxoid, which will protect against type C botulism for about 1 yr. Pet ferrets need not be vaccinated if their food is kept fresh to prevent growth of _Clostridium botulinum_ (Ryland and Gorham 1978).

Ferrets are not susceptible to feline panleukopenia, canine hepatitis, mink virus enteritis, feline rhinotracheitis, or feline calicivirus; therefore, they do not require vaccination against these diseases. Canine parvovirus has not been reported in ferrets, so immunization against it seems unwarranted (Ryland and Bernard 1983).

Anesthesia

Anesthetic agents and recommended dosages are listed in section G.4 of App. 1.

Although a dosage for a xylazine-ketamine mixture is listed, this combination may produce pronounced central nervous system depression and occasionally death. The intraperitoneal administration of pentobarbital also entails a degree of risk.

Surgery

Pet males may be castrated at 6-8 mo of age to reduce agressiveness and desire to roam. The testicles are present in the scrotum only during the breeding season (Ryland and Bernard 1983). Females can be spayed at 6-8 mo of age (Ryland and Gorham 1978).

Scent glands can be removed at the time animals are neutered. Surgical removal of the anal scent glands of ferrets is more tedious than anal sac removal in the dog. The surgical procedure is described in detail in an article by Creed and Kainer (1981).

BACTERIAL DISEASES

Botulism

Ferrets are highly susceptible to botulism type C. Signs of muscular incoordination and stiffness appear in affected ferrets 12-96 hr after eating contaminated raw meat or poultry (Ryland and Bernard 1983). As the disease progresses, they may salivate and will hang limp when picked up. There is no successful treatment.

Tuberculosis

Ferrets are susceptible to avian, bovine, and human strains of _Mycobacterium tuberculosis_. Most animals are infected by consumption of products from diseased poultry. The alimentary tract and abdominal lymph nodes are usually affected (Ryland and Bernard 1983). Tuberculosis may be suspected if an animal has palpably enlarged mesenteric lymph nodes. Outward signs do not appear until later stages of the active infection when the animal becomes emaciated and in some cases develops a paralysis beginning in the hind limbs and progressing to the forelimbs (Symmers and Thomson 1953).

A subcutaneous tuberculin test may aid in diagnosis. A temperature rise indicates a positive reaction.

Proliferative Colitis

Ferrets are among the ever-growing number of species from which _Campylobacter fetus_ has been isolated. Infected animals exhibit protracted diarrhea and dehydration. Mucosal hyperplasia of the colon is a characteristic postmortem finding. Treatment with chloramphenicol or gentamicin and supportive parenteral fluids prolongs the course of the disease but seems to have little effect in reducing eventual mortality (Fox et al. 1982).

Streptococcus zooepidemicus is often the causative organism in pneumonia and metritis (Hammond and Chesterman 1976).

Localized Infections

Staphylococcal and streptococcal infections may cause abscesses arising from injuries to the mouth by bones in the diet or from bite wounds (Ryland and Gorham 1978). Mastitis is frequently caused by *Staphylococcus aureus* (Ryland and Gorham 1978). Vulval infections are common in the female during estrus (Ryland and Gorham 1978).

Treatment of localized infections should follow guidelines established for cats and dogs. However, streptomycin should be used with caution if at all, administering no more than 50 mg within a 12-hr interval, because of its toxicity at higher dosages (Ryland and Gorham 1978). Sulfaquinoxaline is also reported to be toxic to ferrets.

VIRAL DISEASES

Canine Distemper

Ferrets are highly susceptible to canine distemper, and the disease is generally fatal. The incubation period is 7-9 days. The ferret initially loses its appetite then develops a serous to mucopurulent ocular and nasal discharge. The eyelids stick together and affected animals often develop a rash beneath the chin and in the inguinal region. Later, the foot pads swell and become hyperkeratotic. The anus commonly protrudes. The animal's condition deteriorates until death at 2-3 wk following exposure.

Ferrets that survive the catarrhal phase may die in a neurotropic episode with hyperexcitability, excess salivation, muscular tremors, convulsions, and coma. This condition is called the "screaming fits" (Ryland and Gorham 1978).

Treatment is usually unsuccessful. Euthanasia is suggested as a pratical alternative to symptomatic supportive therapy (Ryland and Bernard 1983).

Human Influenza

Ferrets are susceptible to several strains of human influenza virus, which may cause initial signs similar to those of distemper. Within 48 hr of exposure the affected ferret becomes listless, its rectal temperature rises sharply, and it refuses food. Sneezing attacks accompanied by a purulent discharge from the nose may develop. Congestion may be relieved by use of antihistamines. Fever lasts for 1 day and returns on the third day. As soon as the second fever peak subsides, the ferret becomes livelier and soon recovers. Recovery itself differentiates influenza from the early stages of distemper (Ryland and Gorham 1978).

Aleutian Disease

Ferrets are susceptible to the virus of Aleutian disease (AD); however, in contrast to the disease in mink, AD usually progresses slowly in ferrets, with little clinical evidence of illness (Ohshima et al. 1978). Ferrets occasionally become thin; pass black tarry feces, and eventually die (Ryland and Gorham 1978). In such animals the disease is progressive and consistently fatal. There is no treatment, and ferrets with clinical disease should be killed (Williams 1976).

PARASITIC DISEASES

Sarcoptic Mange

Sarcoptes scabiei causes a dermatitis most frequently involving the feet, which become red, swollen, and ulcerated from irritation and chewing (Ryland and Gorham 1978). In some cases a more generalized alopecia and intense pruritis develop (Ryland and Bernard 1983).

Treatment consists of cutting back the claws and removing the scabs after softening them in soapy water. This procedure should be followed by application of sulfur ointment, a lime and sulfur (30%) dip, or other mange remedy. Organophosphate compounds should be used only with great caution (Ryland and Gorham 1978). Corticosteroids (Rx: G.3.d) may be used to reduce pruritis.

Fleas

Fleas are not uncommon in ferrets and, if present, topical preparation used for elimination of fleas in cats are effective and safe.

Ear Mites

Otodectes cyanotis infection causes crusts in the ear canal. Treatment with mineral oil or dog ear mite drugs are effective.

Heartworms

Ferrets are susceptible to infection with *Dirofilaria immitis* and seemingly have little ability to tolerate the presence of adult parasites in the heart without lethal consequences (Miller and Merton 1982). Avermectin derivatives (Rx: G.2.a) have been found effective against *D. immitis* in ferrets (Egerton et al. 1980). No reports of results from administration of drugs more commonly used to treat or prevent heartworm disease in dogs have been found.

Intestinal Parasites

Many types of intestinal parasites have been reported. Identification of the specific parasite is established by fecal examination. Treatment recommended for elimination of intestinal parasites is the same as for cats (Ryland and Bernard 1983).

MYCOTIC DISEASES

Dermatophytosis

Dermatophytosis (ringworm) caused by *Microsporum canis* has been reported in young ferrets and may be transmitted by cats (Hagen and Gorham 1972). Affected ferrets may be treated orally with griseofulvin (Rx: G.1.a).

Systemic Mycoses

Ferrets are susceptible to cryptococcosis (Skulski and Symmers 1954), actinomycosis, and other systemic mycoses, but natural infections are rarely reported.

NUTRITIONAL AND METABOLIC DISEASES

Aplastic Anemia

An aplastic anemia attributable to prolonged estrogenic exposure commonly occurs in female ferrets following a protracted period of estrus (Kociba and Caputo 1981). Clinical examination of affected animals typically reveals pale mucous membranes, swollen vulva, alopecia, petechial hemorrhages, anorexia, and marked depression. Hematologic findings include severe anemia, thrombocytopenia, granulocytopenia, and hypocellularity of the bone marrow.

Since human chorionic gonadotropin (Rx: G.3.a) will cause ovulation and thereby terminate estrus, its use with appropriate supportive therapy would seem a resonable approach to treatment; however, the few reports of successful treatment indicate that ovariohysterectomy and intravenous whole blood transfusions (Rx: G.3.e) may be the most prudent course to follow despite the obvious risk of surgery with a severely anemic patient (Ryland 1982; Ryland and Bernard 1983). Supportive care that includes the use of steroids, force feeding, and vitamin supplementation may improve the chances of survival.

Because of the high incidence of this disease in unmated female ferrets and poor response to even the most vigorous therapy, ovariohysterectomy prior to the first heat period of females not intended for breeding is advisable.

Eclamptogenic Toxemia

Eclamptogenic toxemia usually occurs a few days before whelping. The only characteristic postmortem change is a yellow liver. The disease is thought to be caused by a nutritional inadequacy of some type. It can usually be prevented by addition of uncooked liver to the ration during pregnancy (Ryland and Gorham 1978). Other vitamin and mineral supplements may be equally effective.

Nursing Sickness

Postparturient females may be afflicted with nursing sickness. Signs include anorexia, weight loss, weakness, and muscular incoordination. The cause is thought to be a dietary salt insufficiency, and the problem may be corrected by addition of table salt to the feed (Ryland and Gorham 1978).

Hair Loss

Ferrets are subject to hair loss, particularly if fed a diet containing an excessive amount of raw chicken eggs. This hair loss is due to a biotin deficiency. Molting also occurs as a natural process in response to hormonal influences; females usually molt following the first ovulation of the season, and males molt in October or November (Hammond et al. 1976). At times, ferrets may lose their hair for undetermined reasons. These animals are said to respond to addition of uncooked liver to the diet (Ryland and Gorham 1978)

Steatitis (yellow fat disease) and thiamine deficiencies may result from diets high in fish.

MISCELLANEOUS CONDITIONS

Summer Enteritis

An enteritis of unknown cause occurs in warm weather. Whether this is a specific disease or a syndrome resulting from a variety of causes is unclear. The possibility that *Campylobacter* sp. may be the etiologic agent in at least some of these outbreaks should be considered.

Signs in acute cases include anorexia, bloody diarrhea, and death within 3-4 days. In chronic cases of enteritis, diarrhea may be intermittent and the appetite normal; but the animal fails to digest its food, becomes emaciated, and dies within a month (Ryland and Gorham 1978). Neomycin (Rx: G.1.b) has been used with success in treating the disease.

Zinc Poisoning

Zinc poisoning has been reported in ferrets fed raw meat placed directly on the floor of galvanized cages (Straube and Walden 1981; Straube et al. 1980). Clinical signs of zinc toxicity include muscle tremors, lethargy, and uremia.

Congenital Malformations

High infant mortality is a common problem for ferret breeders. Many of the deaths are due to killing by the females or failure of lactation. Spontaneous congenital malformations, including neuroschisis, gastroschisis (Willis and Barrow 1971), absence of limbs, and corneal dermoids (Ryland and Gorham 1978) are also relatively common.

Neoplasms

Spontaneous neoplasms appear to be uncommon in ferrets; but ovarian leiomas (Cotchin 1980), squamous cell carcinomas (Zwicker and Carlton 1974), adenocarcinomas, lymphosarcomas (Chesterman and Pomerance 1965), and malignant megakaryocytic myelosis (Chowdhury and Shillinger 1982) have been reported.

Other

Reports of anal gland impaction and dental tartar accumulation (Williams 1976), intervertebral disk syndrome (Frederick 1981), urolithiasis (Nguyen et al. 1979), and cataracts (Utroska and Austin 1979) appear in the literature. Guidelines for diagnosis and treatment of these conditions have generally followed those established for domestic cats. Because of the limited systematic studies of ferret diseases, treatment is based largely on extrapolation from knowledge of similar diseases in dogs and cats.

CHAPTER 8

NONHUMAN PRIMATES

As in microbiology and certain other fields, nomenclature and classification of nonhuman primates are subject to periodic change; nevertheless, an individual concerned with the health care or research use of these animals should be able to recognize the more frequently seen species and categorize them correctly because of their differences in biologic characteristics, environmental and nutritional requirements, and disease susceptibility.

Nonhuman primates comprise two suborders: Prosimii and Anthropoidea. Other terms for nonhuman primates include subhuman primates, infrahuman primates, monkeys, and simian primates.

Prosimians

Prosimian primates resemble squirrels or rats more than true monkeys.

The natural diet of prosimians usually consists primarily of insects, but some prefer a fruit diet and some are carnivorous.

Prosimian species include (1) tree shrews, which are the most primitive of the prosimians, sometimes classified as insectivores rather than primates (Whitney and Mulder 1977), and the only prosimians used in any significant number for biomedical research; (2) slow lorises; (3) slender lorises; (4) galagos; and (5) lemurs.

Anthropoidea (Simian Primates)

No single anatomic feature distinguishes simian primates from other animals. Some important characteristics are the presence of a simplex uterus, pectoral mammae, a pendulous penis, scrotal testes, a clavicle, and a hallux (great toe).

The suborder Anthropoidea is divided into five families: New World monkeys, Old World monkeys, lesser apes, great apes, and man.

New World Primates

Marmosets and tamarins are separated from other species of New World primates by some taxonomists, but they will be classified here as New World primates. They are small animals with soft silky hair and long nonprehensile tails. Representative species are pygmy, golden lion, and cotton top marmosets. Female marmosets often give birth to twins or triplets.

Squirrel monkeys (*Saimiri sciureus*) rank second in the number used worldwide for biomedical research (Held 1981a). They are general purpose experimental primates and particularly important in atherosclerosis research. Squirrel monkeys are widely distributed throughout northern South America and Central America. Animals from each geographic area have slightly differing color characteristics. These monkeys breed well in captivity.

Owl monkeys (Aotus trivirgatus) are the only suitable model other than humans currently used for studies of human malaria. They are also of value in studies of viral oncology and are of special importance in vision research because of their unique eye structure. Owl monkeys are native to a wide area throughout Central and South America. They are not as hardy and do not adapt as well to the laboratory as squirrel monkeys.

Cebus monkeys Cebus spp.) are also called capuchins or organ grinder monkeys. Cebus monkeys have been a popular species to keep as pets.

Old World Monkeys

Physical characteristics that serve to distinguish Old World from New World monkeys include the following:

1. Prehensile tails are absent in Old World monkeys, but some New World monkeys have prehensile tails.
2. Ischial callosities are present in some Old World species, but they are absent in New World monkeys.
3. Nasal orifices are close together in Old World monkeys but wider apart in New World monkeys.
4. Cheek pouches are present in some Old World monkeys, but not in New World species.

Rhesus monkeys (Macaca mulatta) are the most popular species of nonhuman primate for research, vaccine production (polio), and drug testing. Most animals used for research and drug testing have been imported, but an effort is being made to expand domestic breeding programs. Because of destruction of their natural habitat as well as religious and political factors, the supply of rhesus monkeys from Africa and India has continually diminished in recent years, and at this time few if any rhesus monkeys can be obtained from those countries.

Cynomolgus monkeys (Macaca fascicularis) are next to the rhesus monkey in importance in biomedical research in the United States (Held 1981a). Cynomolgus monkeys are somewhat more tractable and slightly smaller than the rhesus monkey and currently more readily available for importation.

Mangabeys (Cerocebus spp.) are slender animals with long legs and tails. They are not frequently used in biomedical research.

Patas monkeys (Erythrocebus patas) are large animals with slender bodies and long limbs (Napier and Napier 1967). Although not used in great number, patas monkeys appear to be good subjects for certain types of cardiovascular research (Held 1981a).

Use of African green monkeys (Cercopithecus aethiops) for biomedical purposes has been somewhat inhibited because of its association with an outbreak of Marburg virus disease some years ago (Eyestone 1968).

Of the baboons (Papio cynocephalus), the Savanna or dog-faced babbon is the species generally used in biomedical research. It is found over a wide range in Africa. The baboon is a large, hearty primate that is especially desirable for surgery and reproductive physiology research. There is a marked sexual dimorphism in baboons, adult females weighing about 25 lb and males weighing up to 50 lb.

Lesser Apes

Lesser apes include gibbons (Hylobates spp.) and siamangs (Symphalangus spp.). These animals have long arms and no tail. They are principally fruit and vegetable eaters.

Great Apes

The chimpanzee (*Pan troglodytes*) is the highest form of nonhuman primate used in significant numbers in biomedical research. It is in great demand for testing human infectious hepatitis vaccine and is also used for psychobiologic research. None have been imported into the United States from the wild for several years, but some are available from established U.S. breeding colonies.

Orangutans (*Pongo pygmaeus*), found in Borneo and Sumatra, appear to be approaching extinction (Whitney et al. 1973).

Gorillas (*Gorilla gorilla*) are native to equatorial Africa. In the wild the usual adult weight is 165–400 pounds, but heavier specimens are seen in captivity (Napier and Napier 1967). These primates are too valuable for any form of biomedical research potentially detrimental to their health.

B I O L O G Y

Suitability of Pets

Although the number kept as pets has declined in recent years, some people continue to have pet nonhuman primates. In most cases ownership should be discouraged for the following reasons (Mulder et al. 1977):

1. They have a high potential to be carriers of zoonotic diseases, including hepatitis, tuberculosis, shigellosis, salmonellosis, and herpes B virus.
2. They are virtually impossible to toilet train.
3. Many species are hard to handle, are destructive to property, and have a tendency to bite.
4. Keeping primates as pets constitutes a drain on a limited wild population.

Anatomic Features

One of the most striking features of primates is their great strength and agility. Monkeys weighing 25 lb and up require more than one person to handle them. They are very adept at opening cage doors and escaping.

Rhesus monkeys and some other Old World species have cheek pouches in which they stuff food to be chewed and swallowed later.

Sex skin around the genitals, tail, and thighs of some Old World species is responsive to estrogens. It becomes reddened and swollen during estrus, with maximum swelling just before ovulation. In rhesus monkeys the sex skin has a corrugated appearance, while a smoother swelling is characteristic of baboons.

Ischial callosities are hard keratinized pads seen on the buttocks of some species of Old World primates.

In a number of species, including rhesus monkeys and baboons, the males have large canine teeth. These are vicious weapons and frequently are either extracted or shortened to reduce the danger from bites. For a time, extraction was the more popular approach, but currently the canine teeth are usually cut. The operation consists of cutting the teeth to the level of the incisors, performing a pulpectomy with dental instruments, packing the root canal with dental paste, and capping the pulp cavity with a dental alloy.

Female monkeys have a simplex type uterus, similar to humans. Determining the sex of nonhuman primates is usually simple except in spider monkeys. The female spider monkey has a pendulous labia that resembles a penis but may be recognized by the absence of a urethral opening.

Physiology

Normal physiologic data for representative species are listed in App. 2. These parameters vary to some extent from species to species.

All Old World primates have menstrual bleeding as a feature of their sexual cycle. This is absent in New World species.

Social Behavior

Within the primate order, several different types of social organization exist (Mulder et al. 1977). The most common is that of a troop containing from 20 to 100 animals (baboons and macaques have this type of organization). Within these troops, there is a definite hierarchical arrangement with one male being the dominant animal. Generally, a small number of males come next in the hierarchy; followed by a group of high ranking females; and, finally, a group of low ranking males, females, and younger animals. An animal's rank has a high correlation to the rank of its mother. The hierarchical position of a female in a troop normally remains quite stable, while the position of a male seems to be more transitory with changes in leadership every 4-5 yr (Mulder et al. 1977).

Primates must be reared in a reasonably normal social situation to develop normal behavioral patterns. Hand reared and isolated animals rarely mate and have other behavioral abnormalities.

HUSBANDRY

Housing

The most suitable housing system for nonhuman primates depends on species, use, climatic conditions, and other factors. In research laboratories, animals are ordinarily confined in metal cages with slotted or grid floors. A built-in squeeze design is desirable when animals are to receive frequent injections or blood collection. Arrangements for housing breeding colonies include indoor pens connected to outdoor runs, covered cylindrical enclosures referred to as "corn cribs," outdoor corrals with some form of protection from the elements (rain, cold weather, direct sunlight), and free range on islands.

Feeding Practices

Recently imported primates are frequently undernourished. After capture, they may be held for some time by the trapper before shipment. During this time they usually receive only small amounts of fruits and vegetables; therefore their diet is likely to be deficient in protein. Because of the high level of fruits and starches often fed by owners, pet monkeys also may have protein deficiencies. In this condition, animals are susceptible to pneumonia, bacterial enteritis, and other illnesses.

Most commercially milled pelleted diets adequately meet the nutritional needs of nonhuman primates if fed fresh and deterioration during storage is prevented. Commercial diets prepared for New World monkeys usually contain 25% protein, while Old World monkey diets typically contain 15% protein. A 25% protein diet is recommended by some nutritionists for pregnant, lactating, or growing Old World monkeys.

In addition to providing required nutrients, food that monkeys particularly favor (such as peanut butter, jelly, and fruit juices) offer convenient means of administering medication.

Vitamin C

Most animals can synthesize vitamin C, but primates and guinea pigs require a dietary source. The daily requirement of ascorbic acid is 1-4 mg/kg body weight for maintenance of a vigorous growing animal (Whitney et al. 1973).

Commercial monkey chows usually contain adequate amounts of vitamin C if properly stored and fed within 90 days of milling.

Most pet owners and some laboratories supplement diets with fresh fruits and vegetables. This practice is in most cases not necessary in Old World species if the commercial chow is fresh and palatable, and it adds considerably to the cost of feeding primates. On the other hand, fresh fruit 3-4 times/wk is probably advisable for New World monkeys (Harkness 1982).

Without an adequate dietary supply of vitamin C, typical signs of scurvy develop in nonhuman primates. The usual clinical signs are swelling of the epiphyses of long bones and hemorrhage of the gums, eyes, and periosteum.

To treat animals deficient in vitamin C, administer 25 mg or more per animal per day either orally or parenterally until clinical signs disappear (Whitney 1979).

Vitamin D

A deficiency of vitamin D in a usable form results in metabolic bone disease in primates. This condition is referred to as simian bone disease, cage paralysis, or osteodystrophia fibrosa. Metabolic bone disease also can be due to a calcium deficiency or a calcium-phosphorus imbalance.

New World monkeys cannot utilize vitamin D_2; thus they should be fed a diet containing vitamin D_3, particularly if housed indoors out of the sunlight.

Animals with simian bone disease develop soft bones, kyphosis (humpback), deformities of long bones, multiple fractures, and high levels of serum alkaline phosphatase. Radiographs show thinning of cortical bone.

Correction of the diet including provision of vitamin D in a usable form will prevent further progression of simian bone disease but may not eliminate existing bony deformities.

Pyridoxine

A pyridoxine deficiency may develop after prolonged administration of isoniazid for prevention of tuberculosis.

Signs of pyridoxine deficiency are rather nonspecific and include emaciation, weakness, and occasionally central nervous system (CNS) signs (Whitney et al. 1973).

TECHNIQUES AND MANAGEMENT

Manual Restraint

For animals weighing 15 lb or less, manual restraint is satisfactory.

Leather gloves are recommended for catching unsedated monkeys. Welder's gloves with gauntlets are satisfactory for this purpose.

To catch a monkey, grab it from behind the head or neck with one hand and grasp the legs with the other. After removing the monkey from its cage, an assistant can restrain the animal by grasping its arms between the elbow and the humerus and holding them behind the monkey's back with one hand while holding its feet with the other. The wrist and ankles can be bound with adhesive tape if desired.

Chemical Restraint

For primates weighing 20-25 lb or more, chemical restraint is strongly recommended. Administration of a sedative is greatly facilitated by restraint in a squeeze-back cage.

Ketamine (Rx: H.6.i) is the most popular drug at this time for chemical restraint of primates. Ketamine alone, however, is not satisfactory for major surgery. For this purpose, ketamine should be supplemented with an anesthetic such as pentobarbital or methoxyflurane.

Chimpanzees do not become fully grown until 10 yr or more, but a 20-kg, 4-yr-old chimp has tremendous strength and cannot be safely restrained by two people unless well sedated (Whitney 1979).

A list of general anesthetics, sedatives, and analgesics can be found in section H.6 of App. 1. Local anesthestics are of limited value because of the tendency toward self-mutilation by primates.

Physical Examination

Incoming primates and primate patients should receive thorough physical examinations. Because of the danger of zoonoses, rubber gloves should be worn when examining nonhuman primate patients (Whitney 1979), particularly when examining the mouth.

The examination of a nonhuman primate is performed in a manner similar to a physical examination of other species, with attention given to evidence of diarrhea, nasal or ocular discharge, dyspnea, condition of the skin and hair coat, alertness, and nutritional state. Two areas that should receive particular attention in primates are the lymph nodes and the mouth.

Any enlargement or drainage of superficial lymph nodes is suggestive of tuberculosis and should be noted.

In examining the mouth of a pet monkey, check for dental caries and broken teeth. Ulcers resembling cold sores in the mouth of a macaque are suggestive of herpes B virus, which is of potential danger to humans. Hemorrhage of the gums and gingivitis are characteristic of vitamin C deficiencies (Whitney 1979).

Diagnostic Testing

Various laboratory tests including complete blood counts and fecal bacterial and parasitic examination may be indicated.

The tuberculin skin test is the most practical and reliable method for detecting tuberculosis and is a vital part of the initial examination. The procedure usually employed is the injection of 0.1 ml undiluted mammalian tuberculin (containing 1500 or more tuberculin units) intradermally into the upper eyelid with a 25 to 27-gauge, 1/2 in. needle (Whitney 1979). A separate needle should be used for each monkey. Proper restraint or drug immobilization of the animal is essential to avoid injury to the eyelid. The eyelid is the chosen site because it facilitates reading of the tests without capturing animals again. Tests are read at 24, 48, and 72 hr. A positive reaction may range from mild with only reddening to severe with marked reddening, edema, and occasionally ulceration.

Public Health

One of the primary concerns in managing nonhuman primates is the protection of personnel from zoonotic disease. All animals must be regarded as potential sources of zoonotic disease; and generally the more closely related phylogenetically a species is to humans, the greater the danger.

Some of the important bacterial diseases transmissible to humans are tuberculosis, shigellosis, salmonellosis, melioidosis, and staphylococcal and streptococcal infections.

Among the important viral diseases transmissible to humans from nonhuman primates are herpes B, viral hepatitis, poxviruses (monkeypox, benign epidermal monkeypox, yaba virus, molluscum contagiosum), yellow fever, SV-40 virus, poliomyelitis, rabies, Marburg virus, and measles.

The more important parasitie diseases transmissible from nonhuman primates to humans include malaria and certain protozoan and metazoan parasites such as *Oesophagostomum* spp., *Entamoeba histolytica*, and *Enterobius vermicularis*. Many parasites of Old World monkeys and apes are transmissible to humans, but parasites of New World monkeys are more closely related to those of dogs and rodents (Chitwood 1970).

BACTERIAL DISEASES

Tuberculosis

Tuberculosis is caused by an acid-fast aerobic rod. Nonhuman primates are susceptible to the human, bovine, and avian strains of *Mycobacterium*; however, the human strain is by far the most frequent cause of simian tuberculosis. While not the most common disease of nonhuman primates, it is potentially the most devastating that is likely to be encountered.

All species are capable of contracting tuberculosis, but the disease is more prevalent in some species than others. In over half the cases, initial infection is acquired through the respiratory tract; most of the remaining are the result of intestinal tract invasion (Whitney et al. 1977). Infection can also be acquired through cutaneous infection by such means as bites and tattoo needles. Experimentally induced tuberculosis has been observed to progress from initial infection to death in from 6 wk to 12 mo (Whitney et al. 1977).

The clinical signs of tuberculosis are usually not striking until the disease is in an advanced stage. The most commonly recognized signs are lethargy and weight loss (Whitney et al. 1973). Other clinical signs are pneumonia, diarrhea, skin ulceration, and suppuration of lymph nodes. In some cases no signs of illness are observed, but sudden death occurs in what appeared to be a normal animal.

Yellowish caseous nodules of various size are characteristic of the disease. Lesions are most commonly seen in the lungs and hilar lymph nodes. Other organs frequently involved are the liver; spleen; and lymph nodes of the abdominal, inguinal, and axillary areas.

Classic tubercles have a central zone of caseation necrosis with neutrophils and lymphocytes surrounded by a zone of epithelioid cells. Multinucleated giant cells of Langhan's type may be seen. Mineralization and fibrosis of the tubercles are rare in nonhuman primates.

Diseases from which tuberculosis must be distinguished include lung mites, pulmonary nocardiosis, pseudotuberculosis, systemic mycoses, and neoplasms.

By far the most important tool for detecting tuberculosis is the intradermal tuberculin test. The procedure for performing such a test in a nonhuman primate is described under Management and Techniques. The culturing of blood, sputum, and feces and radiography have a place in the diagnosis of tuberculosis, but none of these alone are dependable or efficient diagnostic techniques. Radiography is of value in detecting advanced anergic cases; however, the lesions of nonhuman primate tuberculosis are often difficult to detect by this means because calcium is rarely deposited in the lesions and the heart blocks lesions around the hilar lymph nodes. Other factors that limit the value of chest radiographs are the small size of early lesions, lack of encapsulation, and the fact that granulomas appear in many organs other than the lungs (Whitney et al. 1977).

The most effective means of control is quarantine, testing, and elimination of reactors. Isoniazid (Rx: H.l.h) may be used to treat or prevent tuberculosis in extremely valuable animals such as the great apes. Its effectiveness may be enhanced by combining with streptomycin or other drugs. Disadvantages of isoniazid are that it (1) may induce resistant strains; (2) may mask the disease, since during treatment clinical signs may be eliminated and an animal may respond negatively to tuberculin tests, although clnical signs reappear after discontinuation of treatment; (3) may produce a pyriodoxine deficiency; and (4) may alter experimental results.

Although elimination of infected animals is currently the preferred means of controlling tuberculosis in a colony, the growing scarcity and increased price of nonhuman primates may lead to greater acceptance of isoniazid and other drugs for prophylaxis and treatment in the future.

Simian tuberculosis poses a significant health hazard for humans. The infection rate in personnel in direct contact with simians is much greater than in the general population (Lennette 1973).

Bacterial Gastroenteritis

The most common health problems of nonhuman primates are bacterial enteritis and bacterial pneumonia. These diseases may be latent in the animal in an unstressed state; but active disease may be precipitated by the stress of transportation, change in diet, and emotional stress of a new location.

The most common cause of bacterial enteritis in primates is shigellosis, most frequently due to _Shigella flexneri_. Shigellosis can be transmitted to caretakers or other personnel who then become carriers of the organisms. Although adults seldom become clinically ill, the disease can be severe or even fatal in children (Whitney 1975).

Although less common than _Shigella_ spp. infections, gastroenteritis from _Salmonella_ spp. infections also occurs in nonhuman primates. Contaminated feed (Orcutt 1980) and contact with infected animals are the principal sources of infection with _Salmonella_ spp. Other enteric pathogens such as _Escherichia coli_ are occasionally incriminated as causes of gastroenteritis.

The clinical signs of shigellosis are depression, weakness, emaciation, and dehydration, with terminal diarrhea that may contain variable amounts of blood and mucus (McClure et al. 1978). Abdominal pain is often evident, and the affected primate may bend forward in a sitting position with its hands folded across its abdomen. Typically, as the disease progresses, the animal becomes semicomatose and lies prostrate in its cage (Carlton and Hunt 1978). Death may occur from 24 hr to 2 wk after onset of illness. The clinical features of _Salmonella_ spp. infection are similar to those of _Shigella_ spp. infection except that vomiting is more common with salmonellosis and the course of the disease is often less acute.

The gross lesions of shigellosis and salmonellosis are not readily distinguishable and the two may exist as a mixed infection (Carlton and Hunt 1978). In fatal cases of shigellosis the colon is usually distended and contains mucus and occasionally blood; the mucosa is thickened, reddened, and may be ulcerated and the surface covered by an exudate composed of fibrin and necrotic cells. Typical gross findings with salmonellosis are pasty to liquid intestinal contents, a swollen and reddened intestinal mucosa, and splenic congestion. With _Salmonella_ spp. infection the ileum is frequently involved while ileal involvement is infrequent with shigellosis (Carlton and Hunt 1978).

Several attempts may be required to recover _Shigella_ organisms from rectal swabs. In culturing for intestinal pathogens, the swab should be inserted past the anal sphincter directly into the rectum and used to scrape the surface of the mucosa. The bacteria are very sensitive to drying; therefore, swabs must be protected before presentation to the laboratory. Ideally, plates are streaked directly from rectal swabs immediately following specimen collection.

Culture and sensitivities are important in selection of the proper antibiotic. Antibiotics commonly used in treating bacterial gastroenteritis include furazolidone (Rx: H.1.e), chloramphenicol (Rx: H.1.d), neomycin (Rx: H.1.1), and trimethoprim (Rx: H.1.r). The combination of trimethoprim and a sulfonamide is effective in treating both the active disease and the carrier state of *Shigella* spp. infections (Orcutt 1980).

Supportive measures are very important in treatment of gastroenteritis in primates. Antisecretory drugs (anticholinergics) such as Biosol-M (Rx: H.5.c) or Lomotil (Rx: H.5.f), and kaolin and pectin (Rx: H.5.j), or other intestinal absorbents are indicated in treating diarrhea. Fluid and electrolyte replacement is essential in cases of severe diarrhea. New World primates particularly need relatively large amounts of fluids. Lactated Ringer's solution is used for fluid replacement (Rx: H.5.k). This may be given subcutaneously for overnight maintenance. Desiccated lactobacillus acidophilous (Rx: H.5.1) is useful in treating chronic cases of diarrhea in nonhuman primates. If New World primates become weak and begin sitting on their buttocks, steps should be taken to prevent formation of decubitus ulcers that may develop because they lack ischial callosities.

Bacterial Pneumonia

Bacterial pneumonia ranks with tuberculosis and dysentery as major causes of death in primate colonies. *Streptococcus* (*Diplococcus*) *pneumoniae* is a common cause of pneumonia in Old World primates (Whitney et al. 1973), while a high incidence of pneumonia from *Bordetella bronchiseptica* has been reported in New World monkeys (Seibold et al. 1970). Other organisms often associated with pneumonia in primates include *Klebsiella pneumoniae*, *Pasteurella multocida*, *Haemophilus influenzae*, *Staphylococcus aureus*, and various Streptococci other than *Streptococcus pneumoniae*.

The clinical signs are those that might be expected with pneumonia-fever, rapid pulse, sneezing, coughing, mucopurulent nasal discharge, lethargy, anorexia, and dyspnea. In severe cases cyanosis and prostration may be evident. The disease course is from several days to several weeks. With *S. pneumoniae*, a meningitis with accompanying CNS signs is a frequent complication.

At necropsy, the lungs are typically consolidated and red to gray in color. A fibrinous pleuritis, pericarditis, and possibly empyema is characteristic of infections with *S. pneumoniae*. A meningitis appears grossly as a diffuse gray opacity of the meninges with an accumulation of yellow-white viscous material in the sulci.

Culture and sensitivities are important in selection of the most effective antibiotic. Penicillin (Rx: H.1.n; H.1.o), tetracycline (Rx: H.1.q), and chloramphenicol (Rx: H.1.d) are most commonly used in treating bacterial pneumonia. Supportive treatment includes maintaining the ambient temperature at a comfortable level and providing nourishment and fluid if animals refuse food and water. Bronchial dilators (Rx: H.5.a) and decongestants (Rx: H.5.g) are often useful (Whitney 1979).

Pseudotuberculosis

Pseudotuberculosis is caused by *Yersinia pseudotuberculosis*. The disease has been reported in both Old World and New World monkeys (Buhles et al. 1981; Rosenberg et al. 1980) and has also been observed in humans. Clinically acute yersiniosis typically occurs as an enteritis primarily affecting the jejunum and ileum.

In its chronic form, lesions may be confused grossly with tuberculosis. Microscopically, a lesion in the liver or lung consists of a central area of necrosis with neutrophils and clumps of bacteria surrounded by a zone of macrophages (Stookey and Moe 1978).

Melioidosis

Melioidosis is caused by *Pseudomonas pseudomallei*. The disease has been reported in Old World monkeys and apes. Humans are susceptible to the disease but direct transmission from nonhuman primates has not been reported.

The clinical course of melioidosis may be acute and fulminant or chronic (Stookey and Moe 1978). Multiple abscesses are seen as swelling in several locations (Carlton and Hunt 1978). Gross findings in the lung typically consist of focal lesions up to 3 cm in diameter surrounded by a red halo (Stookey and Moe 1978).

VIRAL DISEASES

Herpesvirus

Although a large number of herpesviruses have been isolated from different species of nonhuman primates, the pathogenic effects of some of these isolates have not been established. However, a number of specific herpesviruses do produce highly fatal systemic diseases in nonhuman primates. In most herpes infections, there are two types of hosts: a reservoir or natural host in which the virus exists as a subclinical or latent infection and an aberrant or accidental host of a different species in which the infection is usually fatal.

Herpes simplex is the cause of fever blisters in humans. In this disease, humans are the reservoir hosts and certain species of nonhuman primates, primarily marmosets and owl monkeys, are fatally infected. Lesions in affected monkeys are similar to those seen with herpes T, which will be described after herpes B (Hunt and Melendez 1969).

Herpes B (herpes simiae) is of major importance in primate virology. The macaque group of Old World primates, particularly rhesus and cynomolgus monkeys, are the natural hosts for herpes B and humans are one of the aberrant hosts of this virus. The disease is most commonly transmitted to humans by bites and scratches from infected monkeys. Lesions in monkeys usually appear as vesicles or ulcers of the lips, tongue, and cheeks. Monkeys rarely develop a febrile systemic disease or show any serious effects from the virus. The concern is not for monkey health but the danger the disease poses for humans. Even after the oral ulcers have healed, infected monkeys may transmit the disease (Hunt and Melendez 1969).

In humans the disease is seen as an encephalomyelitis. The incidence of disease in humans is very low, with only about 20 cases reported; however, in that number there are only 3 survivors (Hall 1973) and they have had varying degrees of permanent CNS damage (Whitney 1975).

The squirrel monkey is the usual natural host for herpes T (herpesvirus tamarinus); however, it also can exist as a latent infection in cebus and spider monkeys. Fatal infections most commonly occur in owl monkeys and occasionally in tamarins and marmosets. Lesions in fatally infected monkeys include facial swelling with self-mutilation; ulceration of the lips, tongue, and gastrointestinal tract; and hepatic necrosis (Hunt and Melendez 1969).

The natural host of herpesvirus saimiri is the squirrel monkey, and the infection in this species is asymptomatic. If the virus recovered from infected squirrel monkeys is inoculated into owl monkeys or marmosets, it induces a malignant lymphoma and lymphocytic leukemia (Hunt and Melendez 1969).

Measles

Measles (rubeola) is a rather common, usually mild viral disease of macaques and most other species of Old World primates. The New World species appear to be somewhat more resistant to infections; however, this assumption has not been clearly established (Stookey and Moe 1978).

Clinical signs most frequently seen are the presence of a nasal and ocular discharge, conjunctivitis, facial edema, blepharitis, a papular skin rash, and sometimes signs of pneumonia. The pneumonia that occurs is of a giant cell type. Active infection with measles interferes with the response to tuberculin tests (Potkay et al. 1966).

Human measles vaccine (1/2 ml for marmosets and owl monkeys) is reported to be effective in protecting monkeys from the disease. Another important preventive measure is avoiding exposure to infected humans, which are the usual source of monkey infections.

Pox

Five different poxviruses are known to infect nonhuman primates: monkeypox, smallpox, benign epidermal monkeypox (BEMP), yaba, and molluscum contagiosum. All these can infect humans (Douglas et al. 1967; Kupper et al. 1970). In most cases, however, only epidermal changes are seen in humans, with no signs of systemic illness (Eyestone 1968).

Monkeypox is characterized by circular lesions of the skin, which undergo vesiculation and ulceration. Immunization with vaccinia protects both human and nonhuman primates against monkeypox (National Cancer Institute 1979).

BEMP is seen as nonvesiculating pocks with epidermal necrosis. It occurs primarily in macaques.

Yaba is characterized by the presence of nodular subcutaneous lesions that have a tendency to ulcerate.

Molluscum contagiosum is a poxvirus disease primarily of humans; it has also been reported in chimpanzees (Douglas et al. 1967), in which the lesions appear as papular cutaneous elevations.

Treatment of pox lesions, if indicated, should be directed at prevention of self-mutilation and secondary infection through the use of sedatives, antipruritic drugs, steroids, and antibiotics (Johnson et al. 1981).

Hepatitis

People working with chimpanzees are at some risk to human infectious hepatitis. Humans exposed to infected chimpanzees can be protected by immune serum globulin repeated at 6-mo intervals (Krushak 1970).

Poliomyelitis

Chimpanzees, gorillas, and orangutans are susceptible to the virus of human poliomyelitis (Allmond et al. 1967). The clinical signs and lesions are similar to those seen with the disease in humans (Johnson et al. 1981). Susceptible species and people working with these species should be immunized with human polio vaccine.

Rabies

Rabies occurs occasionally in nonhuman primates. If they are vaccinated against rabies, a killed vaccine should be used.

Other Viral Infections

Other viral infections that have been reported in nonhuman primates include yellow fever, chickenpox, simian hemorrhagic fever, and Marburg virus (Johnson et al. 1981).

PARASITIC DISEASE

Protozoa

Entamoeba histolytica is pathogenic for all primates, although it is less pathogenic for monkeys and apes than for humans (Whitney 1979). Special techniques may be needed to recover and identify the organism, which is not ordinarily detected by routine fecal flotation (Johnson et al. 1981). The most common lesions are gut ulceration and hepatic abscesses. Ulcers in the gut typically have a flask shape (McClure et al. 1978).

The recommended treatment is diiodohydroxyquin (Rx: H.3.c) or a 3-wk course of diiodohydroxyquin and a 2-wk course of tetracycline (Rx: H.3.c).

Balantidium coli is frequently found in fecal specimens of various nonhuman primate species, especially the anthropoid apes (McClure et al. 1978). The pathogenicity of the organism for nonhuman primates has not been clearly established, but ulcerative lesions in the large intestine resembling those produced by *Entamoeba histolytica* have been reported (Shadduck and Pakes 1978). Infections in humans may result in severe diarrhea and dysentery (McClure et al. 1978).

The recommended treatment for elimination of *B. coli* is diiodohydroxyquin (Rx: H.3.c).

Both Old World and New World monkeys as well as apes can contract malaria through infection with various species of *Plasmodia*. The disease is usually nonfatal in nonhuman primates but infected animals may serve as a source of infection for humans if the required species of mosquito vectors are present (Shadduck and Pakes 1978). Various species of anopheline mosquitoes transmit malaria.

Nematodes

Nodular worms (*Oesophagostomum* spp.) are the most important metazoan parasites affecting Old World primates (Whitney 1979). The parasite produces firm, smooth black or white nodules in the wall of the colon seen most easily from the serosal surface (Shadduck and Pakes 1978). Both the eggs and the adult worm resemble canine hookworms. Heavy infections may cause diarrhea and adhesions. The treatment of choice is thiabendazole (Rx: H.3.n) administered through a nasogastric catheter. Treatment should be repeated in 2-3 wk.

Strongyloides (*Strongyloides fullbornii*) are very common parasites of nonhuman primates (Whitney et al. 1973). Thiabendazole (Rx: H.3.n) and dithiazanine iodine (Rx: H.3.d) are effective in treating strongyloidosis. Treatment with dithiazanine iodine should be continued for 2 wk.

Adult *Dipetalonema* spp. are very common in the peritoneal cavity of New World monkeys. Microfilaria appear in the blood. Although often found in large numbers, the parasite appears to cause no lesions in the peritoneal cavity (Shadduck and Pakes 1978). Affected animals are usually not treated; but if treatment is desired, drugs used for treating heartworms in dogs are said to be effective (Harkness 1982).

Pinworms (*Enterobius vermicularis*), the common pinworm of humans, are found quite commonly in captive chimpanzees and cross-infection between chimpanzees and humans occurs readily (Sedgwick et al. 1975). Pinworm infections in simian primates are usually not serious but cause perianal pruritus and restlessness; however, heavy infections are occasionally fatal (Holmes et al. 1980). The ova are more readily detected by application of cellophane tape to the perianal area than by fecal flotation (Ruch 1959).

The treatment of choice is pyrvinium pamoate (Rx: H.3.k).

Tapeworms

Hydatid disease seen with some frequency in nonhuman primates, is caused by the larval stage of the dog tapeworm, *Echinococcus granulosa*. Hydatid disease also occurs in several species of domestic animals.

The dwarf tapeworm (*Hymenolepsis nana*) is fairly common in mice but also occurs occasionally in nonhuman primates. It is transmissible to humans and does not require an intermediate host to be infective.

The recommended treatment for *H. nana* is niclosamide (Rx: H.3.h).

Acanthocephalans

Prosthenorchis elegans is the thorny-headed worm of primates. This parasite is commonly found in New World monkeys. The adult burrows deeply into the mucosa of the terminal ileum, causing abscesses and granulomas and occasionally peritonitis.

The cockroach serves as an intermediate host; therefore, control requires their elimination. The use of niclosamide will reduce the population of adult *P. elegans* but will not eliminate all the parasites (Whitney 1979).

Arthropods

The most important arthropod infestation of nonhuman primates is the lung mite, *Pneumonyssus simicola* (Whitney 1979). Pulmonary acariasis is found in virtually all captured wild rhesus monkeys.

In affected animals, pale yellow foci containing the mites are found throughout the lungs. In some cases cavitation is seen. Grossly, the lesions of lung mites may resemble those of tuberculosis. Microscopically, the presence of brown to black pigment and a focal bronchiolitis are characteristic of lung mite infestation. Secondary bacterial bronchopneumonia may develop.

There is no specific treatment for lung mites; but ronnel (Rx: H.3.m) (every other day for 4 treatments, then once weekly for 3 mo) has been found to reduce the number of lesions (Finegold et al. 1968).

Pentastomids

The nymphs of pentastomids (*Armillifer* sp. and others) are often found encysted in the peritoneal cavity of nonhuman primates. Adult pentastomids live in the lungs of large snakes; and monkeys are infected by swallowing food contaminated by snake feces.

There are usually no clinical signs in the intermediate host, but peritonitis following penetration of the intestinal wall by immature stages of a pentastomid has been reported (Whitney and Kruskenberg 1967).

Ectoparasites

Among the external parasites reported in nonhuman primates are *Psorergates simplex* (Lee et al. 1981), *Sarcoptes scabei*, *Demodex* sp., and *Pedicinus* sp. (Johnson et al. 1981). Guidelines for diagnosis and treatment of nonhuman primate ectoparasites are similar to those for dogs and cats. Topical organophosphate insecticides and pyrethrins are effective in treating external parasites (Johnson et al. 1981).

MYCOTIC DISEASES

Dermatophytosis

Ringworm in nonhuman primates is caused by several species of *Microsporum* and *Trichophyton* (Johnson et al. 1981). Systemic treatment using griseofulvin (Rx: H.l.g) rather than topical preparations is suggested for treating ringworm lesions.

Systemic Mycoses

Nocardiosis in nonhuman primates is most commonly seen as a granulomatous disease of the lungs resembling tuberculosis. Nocardiosis can usually be differentiated from tuberculosis by the absence of involvement of the hilar lymph nodes (Johnson et al. 1981).

Moniliasis and aspergillosis rarely occur in animals not previously debilitated from other causes (Johnson et al. 1981).

Natural infection with *Coccidioides immitis* (coccidioidomycosis) is limited to arid portions of the southwestern United States (Johnson et al. 1981).

MISCELLANEOUS CONDITIONS

Acute Gastric Dilatation

Acute gastric dilatation occurs with some frequency in macaques. The exact etiology is unknown, but there is evidence that clostridial organisms are involved. *Clostridium perfringens* is usually isolated from the colon contents of animals dying of bloat; however, the condition has not been reproduced by administration of the organism (Pond et al. 1982). Excessive food and water intake are considered predisposing causes. The condition is most often seen in either greedy animals or animals in which full feeding was resumed after a period of restricted feeding. Most deaths occur at night following the evening feeding.

Usually, gaseous distention of the stomach develops rapidly, and death comes quickly unless the primate is immediately treated. The abdominal distention is extreme and is accompanied by an accumulation of subcutaneous gas, which may give the animal a grotesque appearance. Breathing is shallow and labored due to compression of the lungs. Ingesta may be seen in the oral cavity, but neither frank vomiting or bloody diarrhea are usual features of acute gastric dilatation.

Mortality is high unless the problem is detected early and vigorous treatment instituted promptly. Recommended treatment consists of gastric aspiration with suction continued until peristalsis is resumed. Intravenous saline equivalent to the amount of contents removed from the stomach should then be administered. The use of antibiotics and steroids is also thought to increase the chances of survival.

Bloat in primates is prevented by multiple feedings of small quantities of food plus full access to water (Johnson et al 1981).

Endometriosis

Endometriosis is a condition in which endometrial glands and stroma are found in abnormal locations (most commonly on the serosal surface of pelvic organs). When this tissue appears in the myometrium, the condition is properly termed "adenomyosis."

Endometriosis is quite commonly seen in rhesus monkeys, particularly following hysterotomy. The pathogenesis of this disease in humans and nonhuman primates is unresolved.

Trauma

Bite wounds are the most frequent problems seen in group-housed primates and the wounds are often very extensive. Fighting is most likely to occur during establishment of a social order.

Bandages are difficult if not impossible to keep in place and self-mutilation following injury often poses a problem. Otherwise, treatment is essentially the same as for other species. Primates are susceptible to tetanus and should receive antitoxin after penetrating injuries if they have not been previously immunized.

Dental Diseases

Periodic removal of dental deposits with a scaler is recommended to prevent periodontal disease (Chase and Cooper 1968).

Dental caries are more likely to be seen in pet monkeys fed sweets than in research monkeys (Whitney et al. 1973).

Abscesses of the upper canine teeth are not uncommon in squirrel monkeys (Williams 1976). An abscess typically appears as a swelling in the cheek region (below one eye) that may rupture and drain to the outside. Treatment consists of extraction of the involved tooth and irrigation with an antibacterial solution.

CHAPTER 9

REPTILES

TAXONOMY

The class Reptilia comprises the orders Chelonia, Crocodilia, Squamata, and Rhyncocephalia (Frye 1981). The order Chelonia includes terrestrial tortoises (primarily herbivorous), amphibious freshwater turtles or terrapins (primarily carnivorous), and aquatic marine turtles (omnivorous).

Included in the order Crocodilia are crocodiles, alligators, and caimans.

The order Rhyncocephalia contains only one species, the tuatara (Frye 1981).

Snakes and lizards belong to the order Squamata.

BIOLOGY

Anatomic Features

The chelonian shell consists of the carapace (dorsal shell), which incorporates the ribs and 10 fused thoracolumbar vertebrae and the ventral shell termed the plastron. The bridge joins the carapace and the plastron laterally. The shell accounts for 40-60% of the body weight in most turtles, a factor that should be considered when calculating drug dosages (Setser 1983).

Differentiation of sexes in reptiles on the basis of external appearance is difficult.

In chelonias the plastron is usually flat in the female, and the tail is less developed than in the male. The plastron tends to be concave in the male. There are tubercles on the ventral mandible of male tortoises in some species (Frye 1981).

In crocodilians the adult males are usually larger than the females, and digital palpation of the cloaca will reveal a rigid penis (Setser 1983). In some species, swellings caudal to the eyes are larger in males than in females.

Male snakes and lizards have paired copulatory organs called hemipenes (Marcus 1981). In boas and pythons, spurs on either side of the cloacal vent are larger and more prominent in males than in females (Frye 1981); however, this difference may not be readily discernible and is useful only to those well acquainted with the species concerned (Setser 1983). Sex can be more definitively determined in snakes by measuring the depth of the paracloacal sacs with a lubricated blunt probe — the probe can be inserted to a greater depth in males than in females (Marcus 1981). Care must be exercised when inserting the probe to avoid perforation of the cloaca (Setser 1983).

TECHNIQUES

Blood Collection

Small amounts of blood may be collected from a lizard or turtle by clipping a toenail or from the retrobulbar venous plexus in a lizard following procedures used in collecting blood from laboratory rodents. Blood can also be obtained from the jugular vein or dorsal tail vein of turtles and from the ventral vessels of the tail in lizards and snakes (Walshaw 1983).

Medication

A stomach tube can be used to administer medication and nutrients to reptiles that will not otherwise accept food. The tracheal opening is readily visualized in the mouth of most reptiles and can be easily avoided when inserting a stomach tube (Walshaw 1983).

Suitable sites for intramuscular injection are the muscles on either side of the lumbar spine in lizards and snakes and the triceps muscles in chelonians and lizards. Intramuscular injections in the tail and hind legs should be avoided if possible. An injection should be given between scales rather than directly through a scale in snakes (Walshaw 1983).

NUTRITION AND NUTRITIONAL DISEASES

Feeding Practices

The recommended frequency of feeding depends on a number of factors, including ambient temperature and size and species of the reptiles. A detailed description of recommended feeding practices for reptiles is beyond the scope of this book; but App. 3 presents a list of the preferred diets for various commonly exhibited reptilian species.

Anorexia and Starvation

Failure to eat and improper nutrition are the most frequent causes of death in captive reptiles (Setser 1983). Clinical signs of starvation include sunken eyes, shriveled skin, and protruding bony prominences. Failure to eat may be due to lack of acceptable food for the species, too frequent handling, improper environmental temperature, or various other factors. Stimulation of the appetite may be achieved by offering different foods, elevating the ambient temperature, cleaning the cage, or providing a larger enclosure (pen). If other measures fail, force feeding may be attempted by gently administering highly digestible food items or tube-feeding pureed food or food supplements (e.g., Nutrical).

Vomiting and Regurgitaton

Vomiting and regurgitation are seen especially in snakes and are most frequently due to handling too soon after feeding (Frye 1979). Another cause of vomiting is low ambient temperature, which results in a decrease in digestive activity and leads to putrefaction of ingested food (Frye 1979).

Constipation

Constipation may occur in snakes consuming large amounts of furry rodents or thickly feathered birds or may be related to a lack of exercise (Frye 1979). Treatment consists of orally administered stool softening agents and enemas. Gentle palpation with a milking action is helpful in moving large fecal masses (Frye 1979). Warm water baths are also said to be effective in stimulating defecation (Setser 1983).

Metabolic Bone Disease

Most cases of metabolic bone disease are due to a calcium-phosphorus imbalance (excessive phosphorus and deficiency of calcium in the diet), a dietary deficiency of vitamin D_3, or inadequate sunlight. It commonly occurs in reptiles fed diets of only lean meat or lettuce (Frye 1979). Lesions typically consist of deformities of the shell and/or skeleton and pathologic fractures. Radiography will reveal a thinning of the cortex of long bones (Setser 1983).

Treatment should include correction of the diet and the addition of vitamin and/or mineral supplements.

Hypovitaminosis A

Clinical signs are most commonly seen in young aquatic turtles on a diet consisting primarily of lettuce or muscle meat. A vitamin A deficiency results in palpebral edema, conjunctivitis, and respiratory problems.

Treatment consists of either injectable or oral forms of vitamin A (Rx: I.3.h), correction of the diet, and in severe cases, use of antibiotics and ophthalmic ointments to protect against secondary infection (Frye 1979).

Thiamine Deficiency

A thiamine deficiency is usually associated with consumption of certain species of fish such as smelt and goldfish that have high thiaminase levels. Clinical signs of a thiamine deficiency include emaciation, incoordinator, enteritis, and respiratory distress from pulmonary edema (Marcus 1981).

Affected animals may be treated with injectable thiamine hydrochloride (Rx: I.3.g) and correcting the diet.

Hypovitaminosis E

Steatitis due to a vitamin E deficiency is seen in reptiles fed obese rats or oil-laden species of fish such as mackerel (Frye 1979). Affected animals develop anorexia, and the body fat becomes yellowish brown.

Treatment consists of correction of the diet and parenteral vitamin E (Rx: I.3.j). The dosage listed is empirical, but tocopherol preparations are minimally toxic except in gross overdosages (Frye 1981).

Gout

In most cases gout is caused by feeding a high protein diet, excess organ meat, or water deprivation (Frye 1979). Deposits of uric acid may be evident in various visceral and extravisceral sites. The disease is prevented by proper feeding and watering practices.

Hypoglycemia

Hypoglycemia occurs most frequently in crocodilians, especially American alligators, and is most likely to be seen in the winter and spring (Marcus 1981). Affected animals typically develop mydriasis, tremors, torpor, and loss of righting reflexes (Frye 1981; Marcus 1981).

Appropriate treatment of hypoglycemic animals includes elimination of stress and administration of oral glucose (Rx: I.3.f).

ENVIRONMENTAL DISEASES

Trauma

Nasal or rostral abrasions result from pressing against wire or glass cage surfaces in attempting to escape (Frye 1979). Treatment consists of eliminating the cause (e.g., providing a retreat), gentle cleaning, and application of an antibiotic ointment (Frye 1981).

If live rats or hamsters are not consumed immediately after being placed in a snake's cage, they may attack the snake. This can be avoided by stunning the rodents before placing them in the snake's cage (Frye 1979). Bite wounds can be treated by debridement and use of topical and parenteral antibiotics (Frye 1981).

Shell fractures resulting from trauma are common in chelonians. After debridement, exposed soft tissue should be cleaned and povidone-iodine solution applied. The fractured shell can then be stabilized with various materials such as rapid polymerizing epoxy resins, fiberglass patches impregnated with resin, denture repair material, and hoof repair material. After healing, the repair material should be removed to permit normal shell growth if the animal has not reached its full adult size (Frye 1979).

Excess Heat

Thermal burns may result from contact with heat sources such as lamp bulbs (Frye 1979).

Overheating may result from prolonged exposure to high environmental temperatures.

Blister Disease

Blister disease is a form of cutaneous infection beginning as dermal vesicles that become caseous as the disease progresses. It is caused by excess dampness and poor sanitation.

Treatment consists of bathing the lesions with antiseptic solutions and in severe cases administration of systemic antibiotics such as ampicillin (Rx: I.1.a) or chloramphenicol (Rx: I.1.c).

Shell Plate Sloughing

In captive terrestrial chelonians the horny shell plate may be loosened from the bony bed following exposure to a damp environment for long periods. Bacteria and algae gain entrance and may contribute to further lifting of the shell plate.

The condition can be treated topically with Lugol's solution or 1% copper sulfate (Marcus 1981) or with a petrolatum-based antibiotic ointment (Frye 1981) and improved sanitary practices.

BACTERIAL DISEASES

Infectious Stomatitis

Infectious stomatitis, also referred to as mouth rot and ulcerative stomatitis, is most frequently seen in captive snakes but also occurs in lizards and chelonians. *Aeromonas hydrophila* is the etiologic agent most often cultured (Frye 1979). Affected animals exhibit ulceration of the oral mucosa and presence of a caseous exudate. The disease may progress to a secondary osteomyelitis, pneumonia, and septicemia.

Treatment consists of thoroughly cleaning lesions with hydrogen peroxide, application of povidone-iodine solution, and/or an antibiotic ointment (e.g., gentamicin), systemic antibiotics (e.g., ampicillin Rx: I.1.a) and supportive care (B complex vitamins, vitamin C, parenteral fluids, force feeding). Quarantine of sick animals and disinfection of quarters are important in preventing spread of the disease.

Pneumonia

In reptiles, pneumonia may be caused by *A. hydrophila* and a number of other bacteria. Clinical signs include nasal discharge, open mouth breathing, and wheezing. Affected aquatic turtles may swim with a distinct list caused by lack of aeration and reduced buoyancy in the pneumonic side (Frye 1979).

Bacterial pneumonia may respond to various parenteral antibiotics including tetracycline (Rx: I.1.n) and chloramphenicol (Rx: I.1.c) and to increasing the environmental temperature.

Septicemic Cutaneous Ulcerative Disease

Septicemic cutaneous ulcerative disease (SCUD) is a disease of turtles characterized by lethargy, anorexia, and cutaneous ulceration with both shell and skin involvement. Mortality is high in untreated cases. *Citrobacter freundii* has been incriminated as the etiologic agent, although other microorganisms may also be involved (Jacobson 1981).

Parenteral chloramphenicol (Rx: I.1.c) is the drug of choice for treatment of SCUD.

Abscesses

Abscesses are common in captive reptiles and may occur in subcutaneous locations, in internal organs, in the middle ear (turtles), or under the ocular spectacle shield. A great variety of microorganisms have been isolated from reptilian abscesses.

Treatment consists of incision and removal of abscess contents, flushing with hydrogen peroxide or povidone-iodine solution, and packing with a water soluble antibiotic ointment such as Furacin (Frye 1979). Parenteral antibiotics may also be administered.

Ulcerative Shell Disease

Shell rot and shell "fungus" are other terms for this common disorder of aquatic chelonians. *Beneckea chitinovora* has been incriminated as the etiologic agent (Marcus 1981), but other microorganisms are often isolated from the shell lesions. Clinically, there is initially a blotchy darkening of the shell, progressing to loosening and shedding of the keratized shell plates of the plastron and carapace, and leaving raw ulcers and a brownish yellow film. The lesions may heal, leaving a pitted shell, or animals may die from secondary infections.

The condition is treated by local debridement of the lesions, twice daily application of povidone-iodine, and intramuscular administration of chloramphenicol (Rx: I.1.c). To prevent spread of the disease, affected animals should be isolated and the environment disinfected.

Dermatophilosis

Dermatophilosis is characterized by the presence of hyperkeratotic nodules on the head, body, and extremities of some species of lizards (Marcus 1981). The etiologic agent is *Dermatophilus congolensis*.

Salmonellosis

Numerous serotypes of *Salmonella* have been isolated from reptiles. Infected animals do not usually exhibit overt disease; however, they pose a significant public health hazard (Jacobson 1981). This is particularly true of turtles.

Although treatment with antibiotics such as chloramphenicol (Rx: I.1.c) may be successful, euthanasia is usually a more prudent course to follow.

Mycobacterial Infections

Mycobacterial infections are fairly common in captive reptiles. The infections cause granulomatous lesions in the skin and internal organs, leading to a chronic, debilitating, and eventually fatal disease (Marcus 1981). A zoonotic potential exists with some species of *Mycobacteria*.

Euthanasia of affected animals is usually recommended, although use of an antibiotic effective against gram-negative bacteria such as gentamicin (Rx: I.1.e) is reportedly effective in some cases (Setser 1983).

VIRAL DISEASES

Gray Patch Disease

Gray patch disease is an infection that occurs in green sea turtles and is caused by a herpesvirus. Skin lesions are initially papular but eventually coalesce into patches (Jacobson 1981).

Caiman Pox

Caiman pox is seen as a gray-white, circular, raised skin lesion (Jacobson 1981).

PARASITIC DISEASES

Protozoa

Amebiasis is most commonly seen in snakes and lizards. Infection causes severe hemorrhagic enteritis and hepatic necrosis (Frye 1979). Recommended treatments include metronidazole via stomach tube (Rx: I.2.e) or intramuscular emetine (Rx: I.2.d).

Other protozoan parasites reported include species of *Cryptosporidia*, *Coccidia*, *Trichomonas*, and *Hexamita*.

Trematodes

Flukes are found in almost all wild-bred captive reptiles, particularly snakes (Frye 1979).

Cestodes

Adult tapeworms are commonly found in the gut of many reptiles. Niclosamide (Rx: I.2.f) or bunamide (Rx: I.2.b) are effective when the dosage is tailored to the body weight and physical condition of the patient. Certain larval cestodes, particularly spargana, cause tissue damage in migration. These may produce subcutaneous nodules from which parasites can be removed by surgical excision (Marcus 1977).

Nematodes

Reptiles harbor a great variety of nematode species, most of which inhabit the alimentary tract or the lungs.

Piperazine (Rx: I.2.g) and thiabendazole (Rx: I.2.i) have been used successfully in eliminating roundworms from the gastrointestinal tract.

Mites

The most important mite of reptiles is *Ophionyssus natricis*, which is seen most frequently in snakes and occasionally in lizards (Marcus 1981). These mites cause debilitation of the host through exsanguination and transmit *Aeromonas hydrophila* (Marcus 1981).

A convenient means of eliminating mites is the use of dichlorvos-impregnated plastic pest strips (Rx: I.2.a). Providing a water dish in which a snake can submerge itself has also been found an effective means of eliminating mites if accompanied by thorough cleaning of the cage (Setser 1983).

Ticks

Ticks are commonly found on terrestrial reptiles. Treatment consists of manual removal and application of povidone-iodine solution. Pyrethrin sprays may be effective in elimination of small ticks; however, whole body immersion in a pyrethrin solution should be avoided (Setser 1983).

MYCOTIC DISEASES

Sites of Infection

Fungal infections may be seen in the form of pneumonia, enteritis, stomach ulcers, keratitis, dermatitis, and granulomas of connective tissue and internal organs. None of these diseases seem to be of major epizootiologic importance.

Treatment

Topical applications of organic iodine ointments and 1% tolnafate cream has reportedly been effective in treatment of several cases. Amphotericin has also been useful (Jacobson 1981).

FURTHER READING

The preceding is a distillation of information published by various authors concerning reptile biology and medicine and is presented merely as an overview. _Biomedical and Surgical Aspects of Captive Reptile Husbandry_ by Fredric L. Frye and _Veterinary Biology and Medicine of Captive Amphibians and Reptiles_ by Leonard C. Marcus are recommended for those wishing to acquire further knowledge of this subject.

APPENDIX 1

DRUG DOSAGES

Drug dosages for laboratory animals are in many cases based on extrapolation from other species or on empirical observations. Doses recommended by different authors often vary greatly. Caution is suggested where the dosage listed is greatly different from established canine, feline, and human dosages. Although the number of drugs approved for these species is exceedingly small, this is in most cases attributable to the lack of economic incentives for pharmaceutical manufacturers to obtain FDA approval rather than evidence that the substances are ineffective or harmful.

Many of the drugs listed have not been administered by this author; therefore, the efficacy and safety of these dosages have not been personally verified but are presented as a guideline. In general, the optimal dosage is relatively greater per unit of body weight in smaller animals than in larger animals.

The duration of treatment is ordinarily a matter of professional judgment and should be based on such factors as severity of the illness, response of the patient, value of the animal, and degree of stress produced by treatment.

References are given in parentheses following the dosage.

Abbreviations used with suggested drug dosages are:

BW--body weight
sid--once a day
bid--twice a day
tid--three times a day
qid--four times a day
q4h--every 4 hours (q6h every 6 hours, etc.)
TD--total dose
IU--international units
PO--by mouth
IM--intramuscular
IV--intravenous
IP--intraperitoneal
SC--subcutaneous
IPP--intrapleuroperitoneal

A. MICE

1. Antimicrobials

a. Ampicillin--2-10 mg/100 g BW bid (Russell et al. 1981).

b. Chloramphenicol oral suspension--20 mg/100 g BW PO tid; e.g., Chloromycetin palmitate 1-2 drops to an adult mouse tid (Russell et al. 1981) or 100 mg chloramphenicol/200 ml drinking water for 3-5 days (Williams 1976).

c. Gentamicin--0.5 mg/100 g BW IM sid; e.g., mix 0.1 ml gentamicin with 0.9 ml water and give 0.03 ml of dilution to an adult 30-g mouse (Russell et el. 1981), or give 40-80 mg/kg BW SC sid for 14 days (McDougall et al. 1967).

d. Griseofulvin--25 mg/100 g BW PO once every 10 days (Russell et al. 1981).

e. Neomycin--10 g/gal drinking water for 5 days (5 ml Biosol/100 ml water) then use one-half this dose for 5 more days (Russell et al. 1981) or 2 mg active ingredient/ml drinking water for 7 days (Barthold 1980).

f. Oxytetracycline--400 mg (2 level tsp Cosa-Terramycin)/L drinking water can be given continuously or intermittently (Williams 1976).

g. Penicillin--100,000 IU/kg BW IM bid, e.g., 0.1 ml IM bid to adult mouse; avoid use of procaine penicillin (Russell et al. 1981).

h. Sulfamethazine 12 1/2%--dilute 1 ml with 49 ml water and give 0.5 ml diluted solution to 30-g mouse bid or 5 ml/pt in drinking water (Russell et al. 1981).

i. Tetracycline--3-5 mg/ml in drinking water (Harkness and Wagner 1977) or 1 mg/ml in drinking water for 7 days (Barthold 1980).

j. Tylosin--0.2-0.8 mg/100 g BW IM bid or 10 mg/100 g BW PO (Russell et al. 1981).

2. Parasiticides

a. Dichlorvos--0.5 mg/g food for 3 days (Williams 1976).

b. Dimetridazole (Emytryl)--1 g/L drinking water for 2 wk (Frost 1977).

c. Dithiazanine iodide--0.1 mg/g food for 7 days (Williams 1976).

d. Mebendazole (Telmin)--40 mg/kg BW as a drench, repeat in 7 days (Russell et al. 1981).

e. Niclosamide--10 mg/100 g BW PO, repeat in 2 wk (Russell et al. 1981), or 500 mg/150 g ground feed for 1 wk (Williams 1976).

f. Piperazine adipate--4-7 mg/ml drinking water for 3-10 days (Williams 1976)--or piperazine citrate--200 mg/kg BW/day in drinking water for 7 consecutive days, off 7 days, then repeated another 7 days (Hoag 1961).

g. Pyrivinium pamoate--0.8 mg/L drinking water or 1.6 mg/g food for 30 days (Williams 1976).

h. Thiabendazole (Mintezol)--100 mg/kg BW PO once weekly for 4 wk (Burke 1979).

i. Trichlorfon--1.75 g/L drinking water with 1 g sugar to mask the taste for 14 consecutive days (Simmons et al. 1965).

3. Other Drugs

a. Acidification of drinking water--3.0 ml 1.0 N hydrochloric acid/pt drinking water (Russell et al. 1981).

b. Chlorination of drinking water--1.5 ml 5.25% sodium hypochlorite solution (Clorox)/2 gal drinking water; provides 10 ppm free chlorine (Russell et al. 1981).

Acidified or chlorinated water may be used continuously for an indefinite period to prevent *Pseudomonas aeruginosa* septicemia.

4. Anesthetics, Sedatives and Analgesics

a. Chlorpromazine--3-35 mg/kg BW IM for sedation (Hughes 1981).

b. Droperidol-fentanyl--0.02-0.03 ml/g BW IM for sedation; 0.05 ml/g BW IM for anesthesia (Hughes 1981).

c. Ether to effect for anesthesia (Williams 1976).

d. Ketamine--22 mg/kg BW IM for sedation; 400 mg/kg BW IM for anesthesia (Hughes 1981).

e. Meperidine--60 mg/kg BW IM for analgesia (Hughes 1981).

f. Methoxyflurane to effect for anesthesia (Williams 1976).

g. Pentobarbital sodium--40-70 mg/kg BW IV or 40-80 mg/kg BW IP for anesthesia (Hughes 1981).

h. Thiopental--25 mg/kg BW IV for anesthesia (Hughes 1981) or 50 mg/kg BW IP (Williams 1976).

B. R A T S

1. Antimicrobials

a. Ampicillin--2-10 mg/100 g BW PO bid, e.g., Totacillin (100 mg/tsp) 0.25 ml for adult rat bid (Russell et al. 1981).

b. Chloramphenicol palmitate--20 mg/100 g BW PO tid (Russell et al. 1981).

c. Gentamicin--0.5 mg/100 g BW IM sid (Russell et at. 1981).

d. Griseofulvin--25 mg/100 g BW PO once every 10 days (Russell et al. 1981).

e. Neomycin--10 g/gal drinking water for 5 days, then half this dose for another 5 days (Russell et al. 1981).

f. Oxytetracycline 400 mg/L drinking water, e.g., 2 level tsp Cosa-Terramycin/L drinking water (Williams 1976).

g. Penicillin 100,000 IU/kg BW IM bid or 0.25 ml IM bid to an adult rat (Russell et al. 1981) or oral penicillin 15,000 IU/20 ml drinking water (Williams 1976).

h. Sulfamethazine 12 1/2%--5 ml/pt drinking water (Russell et al. 1981).

i. Tetracycline hydrochloride--450-643 mg/L drinking water (Melby and Altman 1976).

j. Tylosin--0.2-0.8 mg/100 g BW IM bid or 10 mg/100 g BW PO (Russell et al. 1981).

2. Parasiticides

a. Dichlorvos--500 mg active ingredient/kg food for 1 day (Wagner 1970).

b. Methyridine--125 mg/kg BW SC (Weisbroth and Scher 1971) or 200 mg/kg BW IP (Peardon et al. 1966) or 100 mg/kg BW SC (Williams 1976).

c. Niclosamide--100 mg/kg BW for 1 wk (Williams 1976) or 10 mg/100 gm BW as a drench; repeat in 2 wk or use 1 mg/g feed for 2 wk separated by 1 wk (Russell et al. 1981).

d. Nitrofurantoin (Furadantin)--0.2% in feed for 6-8 wk (Chapman 1964; Russell et al. 1981).

e. Piperazine adipate--250 mg/50 to 60-g rat in drinking water over course of 3 days (Habermann and Williams 1957), or 200 mg/100 ml drinking water (Rossoff 1974).

f. Piperazine citrate--3 g/L drinking water for 7 days, off 7 days, repeat another 7 days (Hsu 1979).

g. Pyrivinium pamoate (Povan)--3 mg/L drinking water (0.003%) or 12 mg/kg food (0.012%) for 30 days (Blair and Thompson 1969; Williams 1976).

h. Thiabendazole--200 mg/kg BW PO for 5 days (Rossoff 1974).

i. Quinacrine hydrochloride--75 mg/kg BW PO TD (Balazs et al. 1962; Hsu 1979).

3. Other Drugs

a. Acidification of drinking water--3.0 ml 1.0 N hydrochloric acid/pt drinking water (Russell et al. 1981). (See A.3, a and b.)

b. Atropine (preanesthetic)--0.04 mg/kg BW IM (Weisbroth and Fudens 1972) or 1-5 mg/kg BW SC (Rossoff 1974).

c. Chlorination of drinking water--1.5 ml 5.25% sodium hypochlorite solution (Clorox)/2 gal drinking water to provide 10 ppm. free chlorine (Russell et al. 1981). (See A.3, a and b.)

d. Cortisone--0.25-1.25 mg/day SC, IM, PO (Rossoff 1974).

e. Oxytocin--1 unit IM, SC TD (Rossoff 1974).

4. Anesthetics, Sedatives, and Analgesics

a. Chlorpromazine--1-20 mg/kg BW IM for sedation (Hughes 1981).

b. Droperidol-fentanyl--0.13-0.16 ml/kg BW IM for sedation; 0.3 ml/kg BW IM for anesthesia (Hughes 1981).

c. Ketamine 22 mg/kg BW IM for sedation; 44 mg/kg BW IM for anesthesia (Hughes 1981).

d. Ketamine-xylazine combination--80 mg/kg BW ketamine IP and 12 mg/kg BW xylazine IP for sedation and relaxation (Green et al. 1981).

e. Meperidine--44 mg/kg BW IM for analgesia (Hughes 1981).

f. Methoxyflurane to effect for anesthesia (Williams 1976).

g. Morphine--1.5-6 mg/kg BW SC for analgesia (Randall and Selitto 1957) or 5 mg/kg BW SC for analgesia (Lumb and Jones 1973).

h. Pentobarbital--25-40 mg/kg BW IP for anesthesia (Hughes 1981).

i. Thiopental--25-48 mg/kg BW IP for anesthesia (Hughes 1981).

C. GERBILS

1. Antimicrobials

a. Chloramphenicol--50 mg/60 ml drinking water for 2 wk (Williams 1976).

b. Gentamicin--0.5 mg/100 g BW IM sid (Russell et al. 1981).

c. Oxytetracycline--800 mg/L drinking water, e.g., 4 level tsp Cosa-Terramycin/L drinking water (Williams 1976).

d. Tetracycline--250 mg/100 ml drinking water for 14 days (Williams 1976) or 2 mg/100 g BW PO, IM (Clifford 1973).

2. Parasiticides

a. Piperazine--20-60 mg/100 g BW PO; use 3-5 mg/ml drinking water for 7 days, stop 7 days, then treat 7 more days (Russell et al. 1981).

b. Niclosamide--1 mg/10 g BW PO (Burke 1979).

3. Other Drugs

a. Atropine--1-2 mg IP TD (Marston 1976).

4. Anesthetics and Sedatives

a. Ketamine--10 mg/100 g BW IM for immobilization; 20 mg/100 g BW IM for light anesthesia (Williams 1976).

b. Methoxyflurane-ketamine combination--10 mg/100 g BW ketamine IM with methoxyflurane via nose cone for anesthesia (Williams 1976) or ketamine 44 mg/kg BW IM followed by methoxyflurane for anesthesia (Smith and Kaplan 1974).

c. Pentobarbital (60 mg/ml)--0.01 ml/10 g BW IP not to exceed 0.1 ml for anesthesia (Marston 1976).

D. H A M S T E R S

1. Antimicrobials

a. Cephaloridine--10 mg/kg BW IM bid.

b. Chloramphenicol palmitate--20 mg/100 g BW PO tid (Russell et al. 1981) or 0.2-0.3 ml/animal PO bid (Williams 1976).

c. Dimetridazole--500 mg/L drinking water (Le Regina et al. 1980).

d. Gentamicin--0.5 mg/100 g BW IM sid (Russell et al. 1981).

e. Neomycin (Biosol)--5 ml/100 ml drinking water for 5 days, then half this dose for 5 more days (Russell et al. 1981), or neomycin 500 mg/qt drinking water (Williams 1976), or 10 mg neomycin in 0.25 ml water/40 g animal sid via intragastric administration, or 10 mg neomycin in 0.5 g cheese pellet/40 g animal sid for 5 wk for prophylaxis (Sheffield and Beveridge 1962).

f. Tetracycline hydrochloride--400 mg/L drinking water (Le Regina et al. 1980).

g. Tylosin--0.2-0.8 mg/100 g BW IM bid (Russell et al. 1981).

2. Parasiticides

a. Dimetridazole--1 g/L drinking water for 2 wk (Frost 1977).

b. Niclosamide--500 mg in 150 g food (Williams 1976) or 10 mg/100 g BW PO (Patton 1979).

c. Piperazine--3-5 mg/ml drinking water for 7 days, stop 7 days, treat 7 more days (Russell et al. 1981); or piperazine citrate 10 mg/ml drinking water for 7 days, off 5 days, repeat another 7 days; (Unay and Davis 1980) or piperazine 10 mg/100 g BW PO (Williams 1976).

d. Pyrvinium pamoate--0.8 mg/L drinking water for 30 days (Frost 1977).

e. Ronnel--45 ml 33 1/3% suspension in 250 ml propylene glycol (Burke 1979).

3. Anesthetics

a. Chlorpromazine hydrochloride--0.5 mg/kg BW IM as preanesthetic (Patton 1979).

b. Ketamine--40 mg/kg BW IM for sedation; 100 mg/kg BW IM for anesthesia (Hughes 1981).

c. Ketamine-promazine-aminopentamide (Ketaset Plus)--150 mg/kg BW (by ketamine content) IM for anesthesia (Mulder et al. 1979).

d. Methoxyflurane-ketamine combination--ketamine 44 mg/kg BW IM plus methoxyflurane via nose cone to effect (Williams 1976).

e. Pentobarbital--50-90 mg/kg BW IP for anesthesia (Hughes 1981).

f. Thiopental--20 mg/kg BW IV for anesthesia (Hughes 1981).

E. GUINEA PIGS

1. Antimicrobials

a. Cephaloridine--10-25 mg/kg BW IM sid for 5-7 days (Harkness and Wagner 1977).

b. Chloramphenicol palmitate--50 mg/kg BW PO tid (Russell et al. 1981).

c. Chloramphenicol sodium succinate--10-30 mg/kg BW IM bid (Williams 1976).

d. Griseofulvin--75 mg/kg BW PO sid for 2 wk (Harkness and Wagner 1977).

e. Neomycin--5 mg/300-400 g animal PO bid for 5 days (Farrar and Kent 1965).

f. Oxytetracycline--5 mg/kg BW IM bid (*Merck Veterinary Manual* 1979).

g. Succinylsulfathiazole--0.1% in drinking water (Williams 1976).

h. Sulfamerazine--40 ml 12.5% solution/gal drinking water (Russell et al. 1981).

i. Sulfamethazine (12.5%)--4 ml/500 ml drinking water for 1-2 wk (Williams 1976) or 1.33-4.14 ml/L drinking water (Melby and Altman 1976).

j. Sulfaquinoxaline--0.25-1.0 g/L drinking water for 30 days (Schuckman 1977).

k. Tetracycline hydrochloride--225-350 mg/L drinking water (Melby and Altman 1976).

2. Parasiticides

a. Lime sulfur--1:40 sponged over the body (McDonald and Lavoipierre 1980).

b. Lindane--1% used as a dip (Zajac et al. 1980).

c. Malathion--0.5% used as a dip (Russell et al. 1981).

d. Piperazine adipate--4-7 mg/ml drinking water (Williams 1976).

3. Other Drugs

a. Dextrose 50%--1 ml diluted in 3-5 ml saline IV (Williams 1976).

b. Griseofulvin--1 1/2% in dimethyl sulfoxide applied topically (Post and Saunders 1979).

c. Oxytocin--1 u IM TD (Williams 1976) or 0.2-3.0 u kg BW SC, IM (Harkness and Wagner 1977).

d. Vitamin C--50 mg/day PO or parentally (Williams 1976) or 200 mg/L drinking water maintenance dosage (Harkness and Wagner 1977).

4. Anesthetics, Sedatives, and Analgesics

a. Chlorpromazine--5-10 mg/kg BW IM for sedation (Hughes 1981).

b. Halothane (1%)--to effect for anesthesia (Peters 1981).

c. Ketamine--22-64 mg/kg BW IM for sedation; 44-256 mg/kg BW IM for anesthesia (Hughes 1981).

d. Ketamine-acepromazine--0.2-0.4 ml/kg BW IM of mixture of 100 mg ketamine and 20 mg acepromazine for anesthesia (Peters 1981).

e. Ketamine-promazine-aminopentamide (Ketaset Plus)--125 mg/kg BW (by ketamine content) IM for anesthesia (Mulder et al. 1979).

f. Ketamine-xylazine--0.4 ml/kg BW IM of mixture of 100 mg ketamine and 14 mg xylazine for anesthesia (Peters 1981).

g. Meperidine--2 mg/kg BW IM for analgesia (Hughes 1981).

h. Methoxyflurane--3% for induction of anesthesia, 1% for maintenance; ketamine 44 mg/kg BW IM can also be used for induction (Peters 1981).

i. Pentobarbital sodium--30 mg/kg BW IP for anesthesia (Hughes 1981).

j. Thiopental--20 mg/kg BW IP for anesthesia (Hughes 1981) or 55 mg/kg BW IP for anesthesia (Peters 1981).

F. RABBITS

1. Antimicrobials

a. Ampicillin--22-44 mg/kg BW in divided doses PO (Russell et al. 1981) or 10-25 mg/kg BW IM q8h (Raphael 1981).

b. Cephalothin--12.5 mg/kg BW IM qid for 6 days (Russell et al. 1981).

c. Chloramphenicol palmitate--50 mg/kg BW PO sid for 5-7 days (Harkness and Wagner 1977) or 750 mg/pt drinking water (Raphael 1981).

d. Chloramphenicol succinate--30 mg/kg BW IM sid for 5-7 days (Harkness and Wagner 1977).

e. Chlortetracycline (Aureomycin)--1 mg/ml active drug in drinking water (Raphael 1981) or 10 g/ton feed (Flatt et al. 1974).

f. Dimetridazole (Emtryl)--0.025% solution prepared using 45 g active ingredient/50 gal drinking water (Williams 1979).

g. Furazolidone (Furoxone)--2.5 g/100 lb feed or 1-2 tsp (200 mg/tsp active ingredient)/pt drinking water (Russell et al. 1981).

h. Gentamicin--4 mg/kg BW IM sid (Russell et al. 1981).

i. Griseofulvin--25 mg/100 g BW PO once every 10 days or 2.5 mg/100 g BW PO for 14 days. For daily dose, mix one 25-mg tablet Fulvicin UF with 10 ml water and give 1 ml suspension/kg BW PO (Russell et al. 1981).

j. Nitrofurazone (Furacin)--100 mg/1000 ml drinking water for long-term therapy (Schuckman 1977) or 9 g/gal drinking water for 5-7 days (Patton 1979).

k. Oxytetracycline (Terramycin)--30-100 mg/kg BW in divided doses PO or 400-1000 mg/L drinking water; e.g., Cosa-Terramycin 2 tsp (500 mg active drug)/pt drinking water, Polyotic 2.5 tsp (500 mg active drug)/pt drinking water, Panmycin Aquadrops 50 mg/kg BW PO bid (Russell et al. 1981) or 50 mg/kg BW IM in 4 divided doses q24h (Raphael 1981).

l. Penicillin G, benzathine and procaine penicillin G (Flocillin)--2 ml/10 lb BW (1ml/2.25 kg) IM, SC every other day (Russell et al. 1981) or 42,000-84,000 IU/kg BW/wk SC (Cunliffe-Beamer and Fox 1981b).

m. Penicillin-dihydrostreptomycin combination (Combiotic)--2 ml IM TD sid (Williams 1976).

n. Penicillin G, procaine--60,000 u/kg BW IM sid (Jaslow et al. 1981).

o. Sulfadimethoxide (e.g., Albon)--75-100 mg/kg BW PO sid for 7 days (Rossoff).

p. Sulfamethazine (Sulmet)--100 mg/kg BW PO, e.g., 5 ml 12 1/2% solution/pt drinking water (Russell et al. 1981).

q. Sulfaquinoxaline--0.05% in drinking water (Patton 1979) or 6 mg/lb BW (13.2 mg/kg) PO for 5-7 days (Williams 1976).

r. Tetracycline--30-100 mg/kg BW in divided doses PO or 400-1000 mg/L drinking water, e.g., 2.5 tsp Polyotic/pt drinking water (Russell et al. 1981) or tetracycline hydrochloride 600-900 mg/L drinking water (Melby and Altman 1976).

2. Parasiticides

a. Amprolium 9.6% (Corid)--1 ml/15 lb BW (1 ml/7 kg BW) PO for 5 days (Williams 1979).

b. Fenbendazole--50 ppm in the food for 5 days (Duwel and Brech 1981).

c. Niclosamide (Yomesan)--150 mg/kg BW PO (Williams 1976).

d. Phenothiazine--1 g/50 g molasses-treated feed (*Merck Veterinary Manual* 1979).

e. Piperazine adipate--0.5 mg/kg BW PO for 2 days (Brooks 1979).

f. Piperazine citrate--100 mg/100 ml drinking water for 1 days (USDA 1976).

g. Piperazine powder--200 mg/kg BW PO (Harkness and Wagner 1977).

h. Thiabendazole--25 mg/kg BW PO (Williams 1976).

3. Other Drugs

a. Atropine sulfate--0.1-3.0 mg/kg BW SC (Harkness 1982) or 1.0-3.0 mg/kg BW SC (Rossoff 1974).

b. Calcium gluconate 10%--5-10 ml PO or 3-5 ml IV (Raphael 1981).

c. Dexamethasone--0.06 mg/100 g BW SC, IM, IV, IP (Schuckman 1977) or 0.125-0.5 mg PO, IM TD (Melby and Altman 1976).

d. Dextrose 50%--2 ml/kg BW (Williams 1976).

e. Human chorionic gonadotropin--20-25 IU in 0.25 ml sterile water IV (Hafez 1970).

f. Oxytocin--0.2-3.0 u/kg BW SC, IM (Harkness and Wagner 1977).

g. Scourvax II (double strength)--0.10 ml/animal PO (Willis and Jensen 1979).

4. Anesthetics, Sedatives, and Analgesics

a. Alpha chloralose--120 mg/kg BW IV for anesthesia (Hughes 1981).

b. Chloral hydrate--200 mg/kg BW IV for anesthesia (Hughes 1981).

c. Diazepam--5-10 mg/kg BW IM as preanesthetic (Biven and Timmons 1974).

d. Droperidol-fentanyl--0.15-0.17 ml/kg BW IM for sedation (Hughes 1981).

e. Ketamine--44 mg/kg BW IM for anesthesia (Hughes 1981).

f. Ketamine-xylazine combination--35 mg/kg BW ketamine IM plus 5 mg/kg BW xylazine IM for anesthesia (White and Holmes 1976).

g. Meperidine--10 mg/kg BW IV for sedation and analgesia (Hughes 1981).

h. Methoxyflurane to effect following premedication with acepromazine--1 mg/kg BW IM for anesthesia (Bivin and Timmons 1974).

i. Methoxyflurane to effect by nasal cone after induction with ketamine--44 mg/kg BW IM (Wass et al. 1974).

j. Pentobarbital--25-40 mg/kg BW IV for anesthesia (Hughes 1981).

k. Propiopromazine--5 mg/kg BW IM as preanesthetic (Bivin and Timmons 1974).

l. Thiopental--20-50 mg/kg BW IV for anesthesia (Hughes 1981).

G. F E R R E T S

1. Antimicrobials

In most cases dosages established for cats are satisfactory.

a. Griseofulvin--25 mg/kg BW PO (Ryland and Gorham 1978).

b. Neomycin--10-20 mg/kg BW PO (Ryland and Gorham 1978).

2. Parasiticides

a. Ivermectin (22-23 dihydroavermectin B1)--1 mg/kg BW SC TD (Egerton et al. 1980).

3. Other Drugs

a. Chorionic gonadotropin--100 IU IM TD (Ryland and Bernard 1983).

b. Cod liver oil--3-5 drops PO sid (Ryland and Gorham 1978).

c. Dexamethasone (Azium)--3 drops/animal PO sid for 7 days (Frederick 1981) or 0.25 mg/kg BW (Ryland 1982).

d. Prednisone (Meticorten)--5 mg/animal sid (Frederick 1981) or 2 mg/kg BW IM (Ryland and Bernard 1983).

e. Whole blood--10 ml IV (Ryland 1982).

4. Anesthetics and Sedatives

a. Ether--0.25 ml/kg BW for anesthesia (Ryland and Gorham 1978).

b. Halothane--via face mask to effect for anesthesia (Ryland and Bernard 1983).

c. Ketamine--10-20 mg/kg BW IM for anesthesia (Williams 1976).

d. Ketamine-acetylpromazine--20-30 mg/kg BW ketamine IM with 0.2-0.35 mg/kg BW acetylpromazine IM for anesthesia (Ryland and Bernard 1983).

e. Ketamine-diazepam--25 mg/kg BW ketamine IM with 2 mg/kg BW diazepam IM for deep sedation to anesthesia (Green et al. 1981).

f. Ketamine-xylazine--25 mg/kg BW ketamine IM with 1 mg/kg BW xylazine IM for anesthesia (Green et al. 1981).

g. Methoxyflurane--via face mask to effect for anesthesia (Ryland and Bernard 1983).

h. Pentobarbital--35 mg/kg BW IP for anesthesia (Ryland and Gorham 1978).

i. Xylazine--1 mg/kg BW IM, SC for restraint (Ryland and Bernard 1983).

H. NONHUMAN PRIMATES

1. Antimicrobials

a. Amphotericin B--0.25-1 mg/kg BW IV sid (Johnson et al. 1981).

b. Ampicillin--20 mg/kg BW PO, IM, IV tid (Johnson et al. 1981).

c. Cephaloridine--11 mg/kg BW IM bid (Melby and Altman 1976).

d. Chloramphenicol--50-100 mg/kg BW IV, SC, PO tid (Johnson et al. 1981).

e. Furazolidone--5-10 mg/kg BW PO (Whitney et al. 1977).

f. Gentamicin--2-4 mg/kg BW PO bid for 1-2 days then sid (Johnson et al. 1981).

g. Griseofulvin--20 mg/kg BW PO sid or 200 mg/kg BW PO once every 10 days (Johnson et al. 1981).

h. Isoniazid--5 mg/kg BW PO in divided doses (Johnson et al. 1981) or (chimpanzees) 15-25 mg/kg BW PO bid (Fineg et al. 1966).

i. Kanamycin--7.5 mg/kg BW IM bid (Johnson et al. 1981; Williams 1976).

j. Lincomycin--5-10 mg/kg BW IM bid (Williams 1976).

k. Minocycline--4 mg/kg BW PO (Whitney et al. 1977).

l. Neomycin--10-15 mg/kg BW PO (Whitney et al. 1977).

m. Nitrofurantoin--2-4 mg/kg BW IM, IV tid (Johnson et al. 1981).

n. Penicillin, benzathine--40,000 u/kg BW IM every 3 days (Johnson et al. 1981).

o. Penicillin, procaine--20,000 u/kg BW IM bid (Johnson et al. 1981).

p. Sulfisoxazole--150 mg/kg BW PO sid (Johnson et al. 1981).

q. Tetracycline--20 mg/kg BW PO tid (Johnson et al. 1981).

r. Trimethoprim (Tribrissen)--1/2-1 tablet PO bid (Johnson et al. 1981) or 1 ml/9 kg BW SC sid (based on recommended dosage for dogs).

2. Topical Preparations

a. Conofite--bid (Johnson et al. 1981).

b. Forte Topical--bid (Johnson et al. 1981).

c. Panalog--bid (Johnson et al. 1981)

d. Tolnaftate--bid (Johnson et al. 1981).

e. Vitamin A and D ointment--bid (Johnson et al. 1981).

3. Parasiticides

a. Bunamidine--25 mg/kg BW PO (Williams 1976).

b. Dichlorvos--10-15 mg/kg BW PO for 2-3 days (Russell et al. 1981).

c. Diiodohydroxyquin--20 mg/kg BW PO bid for 3 wk (Russell et al. 1981) or 30 mg/kg BW PO for 10 days (Williams 1976) or diiodohydroxyquin 630 mg/animal PO tid plus oxytetracycline 250 mg/animal (chimpanzzee) PO tid (Van Riper et al. 1966).

d. Dithiazanine iodine--10-20 mg/kg BW PO sid for 3-10 days (Russell et al. 1981) or 100 mg active ingredient/12-20 lb BW (5.5-9 kg) with maple syrup bid for 2 wk (Van Riper et al. 1966).

e. Levamisole hydrochloride--5 mg/kg BW PO, repeat in 3 wk (Russell et al. 1981).

f. Mebendazole (Telmin)--3-5 mg/kg BW PO (Russell et al. 1981).

g. Metronidazole (Flagy)--35-50 mg/kg BW PO bid for 10 days.

h. Niclosamide--30 mg/kg BW PO, repeat in 2-3 wk (Russell et al. 1981) or 140 mg/kg BW PO (Williams 1976).

i. Paromomycin--50 mg/kg BW PO in 3 divided doses sid for 10 days (Williams 1976).

j. Piperazine--65 mg/kg BW PO sid for 10 days (Russell et al. 1981).

k. Pyrvinium pamoate--5 mg/kg BW PO every 6 mo (Cummins et al. 1973).

l. Quinacrine--10 mg/kg BW PO tid every 10 days (Russell et al. 1981).

m. Ronnel--55 mg/kg BW PO every other day for 4 treatments, then once weekly for 3 mo (Finegold et al. 1968).

n. Thiabendazole (Mintezole)--75-100 mg/kg BW PO, repeat in 3 wk (Russell et al. 1981).

4. Vitamins and Food Supplements

a. Ascorbic acid--4 mg/kg BW PO (*Merck Veterinary Manual* 1979).

b. Chewable children's multivitamins--1 tablet PO sid (Russell et al. 1981).

c. Cod liver oil--1/4 tsp PO sid (Johnson et al. 1981).

d. Pyridoxine hydrochloride--3.5 mg/kg incorporated in diet and fed continuously during isoniazid administration (Koehn 1966).

e. Tone--6500 IU D_3/lb BW/day PO (Johnson et al. 1981).

f. Vitamin D_3--2000 IU/kg BW in diet (Whitney 1979).

5. Other Drugs

a. Aminophylline--25-100 mg/animal PO bid (Johnson et al. 1981).

b. Atropine--0.04 mg/kg BW IM, IV, SC (Melby and Altman 1976) or 0.1 mg/kg BW IM (Martin et al. 1972).

c. Biosol M--20 mg/kg BW q6h PO (Johnson et al. 1981).

d. Chlorpheniramine--0.5 mg/kg BW/day PO in divided doses (Johnson et al. 1981).

e. Dexamethazone--not more than 2 mg/kg BW IV, IM, PO (Johnson et al. 1981).

f. Diphenoxylate hydrochloride with atropine sulfate (Lomotil)--1 ml/animal PO tid.

g. Ephedrine--12 mg PO q4h (Johnson et al. 1981).

h. Furosemide--2 mg/kg BW PO (Johnson et al. 1981).

i. Hyperimmune human serum--0.33 ml/kg BW IM (Whitney et al. 1977).

j. Kaolin and pectin--1/2-1 ml/kg BW PO q2-6h (Johnson et al. 1981).

k. Lacated Ringer's solution--20-40 ml/kg BW IV, IP, SC (Whitney et al. 1977).

l. Lactobacillus acidophilus--1/2 tsp in water PO sid for 3 days (Whitney et al. 1973).

m. Mucomist--50-60 ml/hr for 30-60 min via inhalation bid (Johnson et al. 1981).

n. Neosynephrine--intranasally qid (Johnson et al. 1981).

o. Trimeprazine--1-2 mg PO qid (Johnson et al. 1981).

6. Anesthetics, Sedatives and Analgesics

a. Acetaminophen--5-10 mg/kg BW PO (Johnson et al. 1981).

b. Acetylpromazine maleate--0.5-1 mg/kg BW IM, SC, PO (Johnson et al. 1981).

c. Acetylsalicylic acid--10-20 mg/kg q6h PO (Johnson et al. 1981).

d. Chlorpromazine--1-6 mg/kg BW IM, PO (Johnson et al. 1981).

e. Droperidol-fentanyl (Innovar-vet)--1 ml/10-20 kg BW IV, IM (Johnson et al. 1981) or 0.11 ml/kg BW IM for anesthesia (Hughes 1981).

f. Halothane with 50% oxygen-50% nitrous oxide mixture--1-4% concentration for induction of anesthesia, 0.5-2% concentration for maintenance (Johnson et al. 1981).

g. Ketamine--10 mg/kg BW IM with diazepam 7.5 mg/kg BW IM for anesthesia (Woolfson et al. 1980).

h. Ketamine--11 mg/kg IM with xylazine 0.5 mg/kg BW IM in combination (White and Cummings 1979).

i. Ketamine hydrochloride--10-40 mg/kg BW IM (Johnson et al. 1981; Martin et al. 1972) or 8.3-13.8 mg/kg BW IM for anesthesia (Kuhn and Arko 1974).

j. Meperidine--11 mg/kg BW IM for sedation (Clifford 1971) or 2-10 mg/kg BW for sedation (Hughes 1981).

k. Meprobamate--100-400 mg/kg BW PO (Johnson et al. 1981).

l. Pentazocine--1.5-3 mg/kg BW (not to exceed 60 mg) IM, SC (Johnson et al. 1981).

m. Pentobarbital sodium--20-33 mg/kg BW IV for anesthesia (Hughes 1981).

n. Phencyclidine (Sernylan)--0.25-5 mg/kg BW IM (Vondruska 1965) or 0.8-1.5 mg/kg BW IM for anesthesia (Johnson et al. 1981).

o. Thiamylal sodium--25 mg/kg BW or to effect IV (Johnson et al. 1981).

p. Thiopental sodium--22-25 mg/kg BW IV for anesthesia (Hughes 1981).

I. REPTILES

1. Antimicrobials

a. Ampicillin trihydrate (Polyflex)--3-6 mg/kg BW IM, SC sid, bid (Frye 1981).

b. Benzathine penicillin G with procaine penicillin (Flocillin)--10,000 u total penicillin activity/kg BW IM at 24 to 72 hr intervals (Frye 1981).

c. Chloramphenicol (Chloromycetin succinate)--10-15 mg/kg BW IV, IM in divided doses bid, qid (Frye 1981).

d. Furazolidone (Furoxone Suspension)--25-40 mg/kg BW PO sid (Frye 1981).

e. Gentamicin sulfate (Gentocin)--2.5 mg/kg BW q72h for 3 treatments or more combined with carbenicillin 400 mg/kg BW sid 9 days (Jacobson 1981) or 2.5 mg/kg BW q72h for snakes and 10 mg/kg BW q48h for turtles (Bush et al. 1980).

f. Kanamycin sulfate (Kantrex)--10-15 mg/kg BW IV, IM, IP bid, sid (Frye 1981).

g. Lincomycin (Lincocin)--6 mg/kg BW IM bid, sid (Frye 1981).

h. Oxytetracycline hydrochloride (Liquamycin)--6-10 mg/kg BW IV, IM sid (Frye 1981).

i. Potassium penicillin G injectable--10,000-20,000--u/kg BW IM, SC tid or qid (Frye 1981).

j. Streptomycin sulfate injectable U.S.P.--10 mg/kg BW IM bid (Frye 1981).

k. Sulfadimethoxide (Bactrovet)--90 mg/kg BW IV, IM sid first day; 45 mg/kg BW sid second through sixth day (Frye 1981).

l. Sulfamethazine solution--0.5 g/kg BW PO sid first day, 0.25 g/kg BW second through fourth day (Frye 1981).

m. Sulfaquinoxyline solution--0.04% in drinking water 3-5 days (Frye 1981).

n. Tetracycline--25-50 mg/kg BW PO bid (Marcus 1980).

o. Tylosin--25 mg/kg BW IM, PO sid (Murphy 1973).

2. Parasiticides

a. Vapona pest strip--1 strip/1000 cu. ft. room space (Frye 1981).

b. Bunamidine hydrochloride (Scolaban) 25-50 mg/kg BW PO, not more often than every 2-3 weeks (Frye 1981).

c. Dichlorvos (Task) 12.5 mg/kg BW PO daily for 2 doses (Frye 1981).

d. Emetine hydrochloride injectable USP--0.5 mg/kg BW IM, SC sid, bid for 10 days (Frye 1981).

e. Metronidazole (Flagyl)--275 mg/kg BW PO (Deakins 1972/1973) or 125-275 mg/kg BW PO sid, bid at 7-10 day intervals for chemotherapy; once for prophylaxis (Frye 1981).

f. Niclosamide (Yomesan)--150 mg/kg BW PO (Frye 1981).

g. Piperazine citrate--40-60 mg/kg BW PO (Frye 1981).

h. Tetrachlorethylene--0.2 ml/kg BW PO, not more often than once a month (Frye 1981).

i. Thiabendazole (Thibenzole)--50 mg/kg BW PO as necessary (Frye 1981).

3. Other Drugs

a. Aminophylline USP--2-4 mg/kg BW IM or suppository as needed (Frye 1981).

b. Atropine sulfate injectable--0.04 mg/kg BW IM, IV, SC, PO as needed (Frye 1981).

c. Calcium gluconate injectable USP--500 mg/kg BW IV, IM in divided doses as needed (Frye 1981).

d. Dexamethasone (Azium)--0.0625-0.125 IV, IM as needed (Frye 1981).

e. Furosemide (Lasix)--5 mg/kg BW IV, IM as needed sid, bid (Frye 1981).

f. Glucose--3 g/kg BW PO (Frye 1981).

g. Thiamine hydrochloride--1.5 mg/kg BW (Frye 1981).

h. Vitamin A (Aquasol-A)--1000-50,000 u IM (Frye 1981).

i. Vitamin B complex--0.5 ml/kg BW IM, IV, SC (Frye 1981).

j. Vitamin E--50-100 mg/kg BW IM (Frye 1979).

4. Anesthetics and Sedatives

a. Acepromazine maleate--0.1-0.5 mg/kg BW IM as required for tranquilization (Frye 1981).

b. Pentobarbital sodium
   1) Turtles--16 mg/kg BW IV, IC IP (Young and Kaplan 1960) or 32 mg/kg BW IP (Kaplan 1963).
   2) American alligator--3.5-4.0 mg/lb (7.7-8.8 mg/kg) BW IM for immobilization (Brisbin 1966).
   3) Snakes--.015-.045 mg/g (15-45 mg/kg) BW IPP (Karlstrom and Cook 1955) for anesthesia.

c. Chlorpromazine-pentobarbital
   1) Red-eared turtle, chlorpromazine hydrochloride 10 mg/kg BW IM followed by pentobarbital sodium 10 mg/kg BW IC 10 min later for anesthesia (Young and Kaplan 1960).

d. Thiamylbarbiturate sodium (Surital)
   1) Water snake--30 mg/kg BW IPP, using concentration of 2-5 mg/ml for anesthesia (Betz 1962).

e. Thiopental sodium (Pentothal)
   1) Water snake--.011-.025 mg/g (11-25 mg/kg) BW IPP for anesthesia (Karlstrom and Cook 1955).

f. M-99 (Etorphine M-99)
   1) Turtles (average 1.82 kg)--0.5-5 mg IM TD for immobilization (Wallach 1969).
   2) Snakes (various spp.)--10-5000 mg/kg BW IM, IPP produced no significant effect (Hinich et al. 1969) or 2.0-15 mg IM, IP TD for immobilization (Wallach and Hoessle 1970).

g. Tiletamine hydrochloride and arylcycloalkylamine (CI-744)
   1) Turtles--3.5-14 mg/kg BW IM for chemical restraint (Gray et al. 1974).

2) Snakes--35-210 mg/kg BW IM for chemical restraint (Gray et al. 1974).

h. Tricaine methane-sulfonate (MS-222)
  1) American alligators--40-45 mg/lb (88-99 mg/kg) BW IM for immobilization (Brisbin 1966).
  2) Snakes--.78-.272 mg/g (178-272 mg/kg) BW IPP for anesthesia (Karlstrom and Cook 1955).

i. Ketamine hydrochloride (Ketalar)
  1) Snakes (3.6-4.5 kg)--88-110 mg/kg BW IM for anesthesia (Glenn et al. 1972).
  2) Snakes (0.9 kg or less)--22-44 mg/kg BW IM for anesthesia (Glenn et al. 1972).

APPENDIX 2 NORMAL VALUES

TABLE 2.A. Reproductive Data

Species	Puberty	Breeding age	Estrus cycle	Gestation (days)	Weaning age	Chromosome number (diploid)
Baboon (*Papio*)	3 1/2-6 yr	4-7 yr	29-42 days	154-185	3-8 mo	42
Chimpanzee (*Pan*)	6-10 yr	9-10 yr	32-38 days	210-250	Indefinite in captivity	48
Chinchilla (*Chinchilla chinchilla*)	7-9 mo	7-9 mo	Polyestrous, postpartum breeding, otherwise 28-day cycle	110-128	60 dys	
Ferret (*Mustela putorius furo*)		1 yr	Seasonally polyestrous	40-42	6-8 wk	
Frog (*Rana* sp.)	3 yr					26
Gerbil (*Meriones*)	70-84 days	90-110 days	Polyestrous, 4-7 days	24-26	21 dys	
Guinea Pig (*Cavia porcellus*)	45-70 days	12-14 wk	Polyestrous, 16-19 days	59-70	21-28 dys or when 180 g	64
Hamster (*Mesocricetus* sp.)	45-75 days	6-8 wk	Polyestrous, 3-4 days	15-18	20-25 dys	44
Mink (*Mustela vison*)	8-12 mo	8-12 mo	Monestrous, bred in March, induced ovulation	40-75	6-8 wk	30
Monkey (*Macca mulatta*)	3 yr	4 yr	Polyestrous, 28 days	155-170	4-6 mo	42
Mouse (*Mus musculus*)	35 days	42-56 days	Polyestrous, 4-5 days	19-21	19-28 dys	40
Oppossum (*Didelphus* sp.)	6-8 mo	8-12 mo	Polyestrous, 22-27 days	12-13	10-12 wk	22
Rabbit (*Oryctolagus cuniculus*)	3-8 mo	6-9 mo	Polyestrous, induced ovulation	30-35	6-8 wk	44
Rat (*Rattus norvegicus*)	37-67 days	72-90 days	4-5 days	20-22	21	42

Source: Collins 1972

TABLE 2.B. Physiologic Data

Species	Life span (yr)	Rectal temp.(°F)	Resp. rate/min	Heart rate/min	Water consumption/100 gm BW (ml)	Food consumption/100 gm BW (g)
Baboon (*Papio*)	15-24	98-100	40-65	120-200	...	...
Chimpanzee (*Pan*)	30-40	96-100	35-60	80-150	...	...
Chinchilla (*Chinchilla chinchilla*)	3-5	102-103	45-65	200-350	...	...
Ferret (*Mustela putorius furo*)	5-6	101-102.5	33-36	...	...	...
Frog (*Rana* sp.)	5-6	38-40	...	35-60	...	...
Gerbil (*Meriones*)	2-4	101-103	70-120	260-600	5	10
Guinea Pig (*Cavia porcellus*)	2-5	102-104	110-150	150-160	10	5
Hamster (*Mesocricetus* sp.)	1-3	101-103	35-120	300-500	10	10
Mink (*Mustela vision*)	6-8	102-103	40-70	270-400	...	...
Monkey (*Macaca mulatta*)	15-25	101-102	40-65	150-300	...	...
Mouse (*Mus musculus*)	2-3	98-101	90-220	300-750	15	15
Oppossum (*Didelphus* sp.)	5-7	93-95	35-65	140-220	...	...
Rabbit (*Oryctolagus cuniculus*)	5-13	102-103.5	35-65	120-300	10	5
Rat (*Rattus norvegicus*)	2-4	99.5-100.6	80-110	350-400	10	5

Source: Collins 1972.

TABLE 2.C. Hematological data (36+, 199*, 203#)

Species	RBC (10^6/mm^3)	PCV (Hct.) (%)	Hb (g/dl)	WBC (10^3/mm^3)	Neutrophils (%)	Lymphocytes (%)	Monocytes (%)
Baboon	4-6+	36-40+	10-15+	8-14+	51#	42.7#	2.82#
Chimpanzee	3-7+	38-43+	10-14+	10-14+	42#	51.6#	0.9-1.5#
Ferret	6.8-12.1*	41-52*	14-18*	6-11*	42-65*	35-55*	0-9*
Gerbil	8.3-11.2*	47-60*	14-15*	8-11*	19*	65-87*	0-3*
Guinea pig	4.4-8.2*	37-48*	11-15*	4-10.6*	38*	55*	2.7*
Hamster	5-10*	57-61*	15.5-18*	6.3-8.9*	17-29*	65-81*	1.4*
Mouse	8.6*	45*	14.2*	9.2*	13-20*	70-86*	1.1*
Owl monkey	3.5-7.7#	31-56#	11.9-16#	3.2-28.5#	13-91#	5-80#	1-8#
Rhesus monkey	5-6#	39-43#	11-12.5#	7-13#	20-56#	40-76#	0.5-2#
Squirrel monkey	7.1-10.9#	43-56#	12.9-17#	3.4-14.8#	13-79#	19-82#	0-6#
Rat	7-9.6*	40-54*	11.4-19.2*	6-18*	14-20*	86*	6*
Rabbit	4.3-5.3*	33-44*	10.5-12.7*	8.1-13*	32*	63*	4.1*

Sources: +Collins 1972; *Wechsler 1983; #Whitney et al. 1973.

TABLE 2.D. Biochemical Data

Species	Blood glucose (mg%)	Blood urea nitrogen (mg%)	Total plasma protein (g/100 ml)	Serum glutamic oxaloacetic transaminase (units/100 ml)	Alkaline phosphatase (units)	Serum calcium (mg%)
Baboon	80-95	8-14	6-7	30-45	9-42	9-10
Guinea pig	60-110	8-20	5.2-6.0	...	...	4.5-6.0
Hamster	60-97	10-20	5.9-6.5	...	...	5.0-6.5
Monkey	60-160	11-27	7.2-7.5	30-51	1.0-7.5	10-12
Mouse	75-150	8-20	4.0-6.1	...	...	4.4-8
Rabbit	85-140	5-22	5.5-7.5	...	...	10-20
Rat	50-115	10-20	5.5-6.8	...	...	6-12

Source: Collins 1972.

APPENDIX 3

PREFERRED FOOD OF SELECTED REPTILIAN SPECIES

The source of the information in this appendix is Frye (1982).

SNAKES

1. Boas of many species, pythons, rat snakes, gopher or bull snakes, Old World vipers, and New World pit vipers usually prefer warm-blooded prey such as appropriately sized rodents and birds. Some will also readily attack and consume lizards, particularly juveniles.

2. Garter snakes, water snakes, etc., will usually accept fish, frogs, salamanders, toads, earthworms, slugs, and carrion. Many can be readily induced to accept dead mice if they are first smeared with the mucus of fish or frogs, making them appear to the snake as fish or frogs.

3. Indigo snakes, king snakes, and many racers usually will eat warm-blooded prey as well as poikilotherms such as other snakes and lizards. The indigo snake has a preference for frogs but when hungry will eat almost anything resembling food.

4. The small ring-necked, brown, and worm snakes and their closely related kin usually will confine their diet to small salamanders, earthworms, and very small snakes and lizards.

5. The racers, vine snakes, coachwhips, etc., prefer lizards, although the racers will also eat mice and ground-nesting birds.

6. Some snakes, particularly the king cobra, are almost strictly snake eaters. They will often accept thawed frozen snakes or even old shed snake skins that are stuffed with dead mice.

LIZARDS

1. Horned lizards and some small sand lizards dine almost entirely on ants or termites. Some will accept small crickets or mealworms as substitutes.

2. Night lizards, "worm" lizards, etc., will usually limit their fare to termites or their eggs. Some will also accept small beetle larvae.

3. The common green iguana, most often sold in pet shops, will thrive on dandelion flowers and their leaves, fresh fruit and vegetables, thawed frozen mixed vegetables, occasional crickets or baby mice, cooked eggs, mealworms, and a small amount of commercial dog or cat food.

4. Tegus, gila "monsters," Mexican beaded lizards, and some of the larger tropical skinks thrive on a diet consisting of raw eggs, chopped lean meat, baby mice or Japanese quail chicks, and occasional fruit or fruit puree. A balanced vitamin-mineral supplement is usually administered once or twice weekly by mixing an appropriate amount with the soft foods.

5. Monitors, depending on their size (from a few inches to about 10 feet), will eat much the same diet as tegus, plus larger rodents and birds. Many will readily accept carrion.

6. The geckos of many species are mostly insectivorous; the larger species will also eat baby mice. Many will lap fruit nectar or puree.

7. Fence lizards, many skinks, alligator lizards, anoles, Old World chameleons, etc., usually thrive on a diet of appropriate sized insects, from the tiny wingless or vestigial-winged fruit flies to crickets, grasshoppers, and katydids. Moths can be caught near bright lights after sundown and fed to the lizards the next day.

8. Highly specialized species such as marine iguanas eat only certain varieties of marine algae and kelp. The caiman lizard, with its powerful jaws and flat-cusped teeth, is superbly adapted to a diet of hard-shelled mollusks and gastropods.

CHELONIANS

1. Turtles and terrapins usually will eat earthworms, small whole fish (preferably live), mice, carrion, and green leafy vegetation (pond weed, Elodea, watercress, swiss chard, romaine lettuce, etc.).

2. Tortoises usually thrive on a diet of flowers (particularly those that are brightly colored--red, orange, yellow, green), succulents, cactus, alfalfa leaves and flowers, clover, dandelion flowers and leaves, fruit, squash, and melons. A small amount of wheat bread and or commercial dog food is usually welcome but must not be fed to excess. Many tortoises will hunt for the common brown garden snail, eating the shell as well as the softer parts.

CROCODILIANS

Alligators, crocodiles, caimans, and gavials (gharials) are primarily carnivorous. The first three will accept fish, meat, and fowl; the gavial prefers to eat fish. It is important that some source of natural whole bone tissue is included with the flesh.

REFERENCES

Allmond, B. W., Jr.; Froeschle, J. E.; and Guilloud, N. B. 1967. Paralytic poliomyelitis in large laboratory primates: Virologic investigation and report on the use of oral poliomyelitis virus (OPV) vaccine. Am. J. Epidemiol 85:229-239.

Anver, M. R., and Cohen, B. J. 1979. Lesions associated with aging. In The Laboratory Rat, vol. 1, H. J. Baker, J. R. Lindsey, and S. H. Weisbroth, eds., 377-399. Academic Press, New York.

Arrington, L. R., and Ammerman, C. B. 1969. Water requirements of gerbils. Lab. Anim. Care 19:503-505.

Baker, G. A.; Leader, R. W.; and Gorham, J. R. 1952. Immune response of ferrets to vaccination with egg adapted distemper virus. I. Time of development of resistance to virulent distemper virus. Vet. Med. 47:463-466.

Baker, H. J. 1977. Introduction. In The Laboratory Rat, ACLAM Laboratory Animal Medicine and Science Series, coord. G. L. Van Hoosier, Jr., 3-10. University of Washington, Seattle.

Baker, H. J., and Bivin, W. S. 1977. Biology, husbandry, and research methodology. In The Laboratory Rat, ACLAM Laboratory Animal Medicine and Science Series, coord. G. L. Van Hoosier, Jr., 11-24. University of Washington, Seattle.

Baker, H. J., and Clark, J. D. 1975. Disease. In The Guinea Pig, ACLAM Laboratory Animal Medicine and Science Series, coord. G. L. Van Hoosier, Jr., 27-37. University of Washington, Seattle.

Balazs, T.; Hatch, A. M.; Gregory, E. R. W.; and Grice, H. C. 1962. A comparative study of hymenolepicides in Hymenolepis nana infestation of rats. Can. J. Comp. Med. Vet. Sci. 26:160-162.

Barthold, S. W. 1980. The microbiology of transmissible murine colonic hyperplasia. Lab. Anim. Sci. 30:167-173.

Bartlett, J. G.; Chang, T. W.; Moon, N.; and Onderdonk, A. B. 1978. Antibiotic-induced lethal enterocolitis in hamsters: Studies with eleven agents and evidence to support the pathogenic role of toxin-producing Clostridia. Am. J. Vet. Res. 39:1525-1530.

Betz, T. W. 1962. Surgical anesthesia in reptiles with special reference to the water snake Natrix rhomifera. Copeia 2:284-287.

Bivin, W. S., and Timmons, E. H. 1974. Basic biomethodology. In The Biology of the Laboratory Rabbit, S. H. Weisbroth, R. E. Flatt, and A. L. Kraus, eds., 74-90. Academic Press, New York.

Blair, L. S., and Thompson, P. E. 1969. Effects of pyrvinium pamoate in the ration or drinking water of rats against the pinworm Syphacia muris. Lab. Anim. Care 19:639-643.

Brisbin, I. L., Jr. 1966. Reaction of the American alligator to several immobilizing drugs. Copeia 1:129-130.

Brooks, D. L. 1979. Coccidiosis and other rabbit parasites. Rabbit Health Symposium, Fort Collins, Colo., 1(1).

Buhles, W. C., Jr.; Vanderlip, J. E.; Russell, S. W., et al. 1981. Yersinia pseudotuberculosis infection: Study of epizootic in squirrel monkeys. J. Clin. Microbiol. 13:519-525.

Burke, T. J. 1979. Rats, mice, hamsters, and gerbils. Small Anim. Pract. 9(3):473-486.

Bush, M.; Custer, R. S.; Smeller, J. M.; and Charache, P. 1980. Recommendations for antibiotic therapy in reptiles. In Reproductive Biology and Diseases of Captive Reptiles, J. B. Murphy and J. T. Collins, eds., 223-226. Meseraull Printing, Lawrence, Kans.

Carlton, W. W., and Hunt, R. D. 1978. Bacterial diseases. In Pathology of Laboratory Animals, vol. 2, K. Benirschke, F. M. Garner, and T. C. Jones, eds., 1368-1480. Springer-Verlag, New York.

Carter, G. R.; Whitenack, D. L.; and Julius, L. A. 1969. Natural Tyzzer's disease in Mongolian gerbils (Meriones unguiculatus). Lab. Anim. Care 19:648-651.

Casey, H. W., Ayers, K. M., and Robinson, F. R. 1978. The urinary system. In Pathology of Laboratory Animals, vol. 1, K. Benirshke, F. M. Garner, and T. C. Jones, eds., 116-173. Springer-Verlag, New York.

Cassell, G. H., Lindsey, J. R., Baker, H. J., and Davis, J. K. 1979. Mycoplasmal and rickettsial diseases. In The Laboratory Rat, vol. 1, H. J. Baker, J. R. Lindsey, and S. H. Weisbroth, eds., 243-269. Academic Press, New York.

Chapman, W. H. 1964. The incidence of a nematode, Trichosomoides crassicauda, in the bladder of laboratory rats. Treatment with nitrofurantoin and preliminary report on their influence on urinary calculi and experimental bladder tumors. Invest. Urol. 2:52-57.

Chase, J. E. and Cooper, R. W. 1968. Dental deposits and their control: An important aspect of the preventative medical program for laboratory primates. Lab. Anim. Care 18:186-191.

Chowdhury, K. A., and Shillinger, R. B. 1982. Spontaneous megakaryocytic myelosis in a four-year-old domestic ferret (Mustela furo). Vet. Pathol. 19:561-564.

Chengappa, M. M.; Myers, R. C.; and Carter, G. R. 1980. A streptomycin-dependent live Pasteurella multocida vaccine for the prevention of rabbit pasteurellosis. Lab. Anim. Sci. 30:515-518.

Chesterman, F. C., and Pomerance, A. 1965. Spontaneous neoplasms in ferrets and polecats. J. Path. Bact. 89:529-533.

Chitwood, M. 1970. Comparative relationships of some parasites of man and Old and New World subhuman primates. Lab. Anim. Care 20:389-394.

Clark, J. D. 1975a. Biology and diseases. In The Hamster, ACLAM Laboratory Animal Medicine and Science Series, coord. G. L. Van Hoosier, Jr., 15-31. University of Washington, Seattle.

______. 1975b. Introduction and husbandry. In The Guinea Pig, ACLAM Laboratory Animal Medicine and Science Series, coord. G. L. Van Hoosier, Jr., 3-11. University of Washington, Seattle.

Clark, J. D. and Baker, H. J. 1975a. Biology. In The Guinea Pig, ACLAM Laboratory Animal Medicine and Science Series, coord. G. L. Van Hoosier, Jr., 13-26. University of Washington, Seattle.

______. 1975b. Introduction and husbandry. In The Guinea Pig, ACLAM Laboratory Animal Medicine and Science Series, coord. G. L. Van Hoosier, Jr., 3-11. University of Washington, Seattle.

Clifford, D. H. 1971. Restraint and anesthesia of subhuman primates. In Textbook of Veterinary Anesthesia, L. R. Soma, ed., 385-393. Williams and Wilkins, Baltimore.

Clifford, D. H. 1973. What the practicing veterinarian should know about gerbils. VM/SAC 68:912-918.

Collins, G. R., ed. 1972. Syllabus for the Laboratory Animal Technologist. Publ. 72-2, 440-445. American Association for Laboratory Animal Science, Joliet, Ill.

Cotchin, E. 1980. Smooth-muscle hyperplasia and neoplasia in the ovaries of domestic ferrets (Mustela putorius furo). J. Pathol. 130:169-171.

Creed, J. E., and Kainer, R. A. 1981. Surgical extirpation and related anatomy of anal sacs of the ferret. J. Am. Vet. Med. Assoc. 179:575-577.

Cummins, L. B.; Keeling, M. E.; and McClure, H. M. 1973. Preventive medicine in anthropoids: Parasite control. Lab. Anim. Sci. 23:819-822.

Cunliffe-Beamer, T. L., and Fox, R. R. 1981a. Venereal spirochetosis of rabbits: Description and diagnosis. Lab. Anim. Sci. 31:366-371.

______. 1981b. Venereal spirochetosis of rabbits: Eradication. Lab. Anim. Sci. 31:379-381.

Davis, T. D. 1974. The Mongolian Gerbil. Aeromedical Review, Selected Topics in Laboratory Animal Medicine. vol. 23. Brooks Air Force Base, Tex.

Deakins, D. E. 1972/1973. Diagnosis and treatment of parasites of amphibia and reptiles. Am. Assoc. Zoo Vet. Annu. Proc., 37-46.

Douglas, J. D.; Tanner, K. N.; Prine, J. R.; Van Riper, D. C.; and Derwelis, S. K. 1967. Molluscum contagiosum in chimpanzees. J. Am. Vet. Med. Assoc., 151:901-904.

Duwel, D., and Brech, K. 1981. Control of oxyuriasis in rabbits by fenbendazole. Lab. Anim. 15:101-105.

Egerton, J. R.; Birnbaum, J.; Blair, L. S.; Chabala, J. C.; Conroy, J.; Fisher, M. H.; Mrozih, H.; Ostlind, D. A.; Wilkins, C. A.; and Campbell, W. C. 1980. 22-23-Dihydroavermectin B-1, a new broad-spectrum antiparasitic agent. Br. Vet. J. 136:88-97.

Eyestone, W. H. 1968. Recent developments of zoonoses associated with nonhuman primates. J. Am. Vet. Med. Assoc. 153:1767-1770.

Farrar, W. E., Jr., and Kent, T. H. 1965. Enteritis and coliform bacteremia in guinea pigs given penicillin. Am. J. Pathol., 47:629-642.

Feldman, D. B. 1977. Simplified gastric intubation in the rabbit. Lab. Anim. Sci. 27:1037.

Fineg, J.; Hanly, W. C.; Prine, J. R.; Van Riper, D. C.; and Day, P. W. 1966. Isoniazid therapy in the chimpanzee. Lab. Anim. Care 16:436-446.

Finegold, M. J.; Seaquist, M. E.; and Doherty, M. J. 1968. Treatment of pulmonary acariasis in rhesus monkeys with an organic phosphate. Lab. Anim. Care 18:127-130.

Flatt, R. E. 1974. Bacterial diseases. In The Biology of the Laboratory Rabbit, S. H. Weisbroth, R. E. Flatt, and A. L. Kraus, eds., 193-236. Academic Press, N.Y.

______. 1977a. Introduction and biology. In The Rabbit, ACLAM Laboratory Animal Medicine and Science Series, coord. G. L. Van Hoosier, Jr., 1-6. University of Washington, Seattle.

______. 1977b. Parasitic diseases. In The Rabbit, ACLAM Laboratory Animal Medicine and Science Series, coord. G. L. Van Hoosier, Jr., 23-30. University of Washington, Seattle.

Flatt, R. E.; Weisbroth, S. H.; and Kraus, A. L. 1974. Metabolic, traumatic, mycotic, and miscellaneous diseases of rabbits. In The Biology of the Laboratory Rabbit, S. H. Weisbroth, R. E. Flatt, A. L. Krauss, eds., 435-451. Academic Press, N.Y.

Flynn, R. J. 1973. Parasites of Laboratory Animals. Iowa State University Press, Ames.

Fox, J. G., and Brayton, J. B. 1982. Zoonoses and other human health hazards. In The Mouse in Biomedical Research, vol. 2, H. L. Foster, J. D. Small, and J. G. Fox, eds., 404-423. Academic Press, New York.

Fox, J. G.; Murphy, J. C.; Ackerman, J. I.; Prostak, K. S.; Gallagher, C. A.; and Rambow, V. J. 1982. Proliferative colitis in ferrets. Am. J. Vet. Res. 43:858-864.

Frederick, M. A. 1981. Intervetebral disc syndrome in a domestic ferret. VM/SAC 76:835.

Frost, W. W. 1977. Prevention and Control of Laboratory Animal Disease: A Therapeutic and Prophylactic Compendium. ACLAM Laboratory Animal Medicine and Science Series, coord. G. L. Van Hoosier, Jr. University of Washington, Seattle.

Frye, F. L. 1979. Reptile medicine and husbandry. Small Anim. Pract. 9:415-428.

______. 1981. Biomedical and Surgical Aspects of Captive Reptile Medicine. Veterinary Medicine Publishing, Edwardsville, Kans.

______. 1982. Role of nutrition in the successful maintenance of captive reptiles, II. An update, Speaker's Syllabi, 455-483. 94th Annual Meeting and Scientific Seminar. California Veterinary Medical Association, Los Angeles.

Ganaway, J. R. 1976. Bacterial, mycoplasmal, and rickettsial diseases. In The Biology of the Guinea Pig, J. E. Wagner and P. J. Manning, eds., 121-135. Academic Press, New York.

______. 1982. Bacterial and mycotic diseases of the digestive system. In The Mouse in Biomedical Research, vol. 2, H. L. Foster, J. D. Small, and J. G. Fox, eds., 1-20. Academic Press, New York.

Glenn, J. L.; Straight, R.; and Snyder, C. C. 1972. Clinical use of ketamine hydrochloride as an anesthetic agent for snakes. Am. J. Vet. Res. 33:1901-1903.

Golden, J. G.; Hughes, H. C.; and Lang, C. M. 1980. Experimental toxemia in the pregnant guinea pig (Cavia porcellus). Lab. Anim. Sci. 30:174-179.

Gray, C. W.; Bush, M.; and Beck, C. C. 1974. Clinical experience using CI-744 in chemical restraint and anesthesia of exotic specimens. J. Zoo Anim. Med. 5(4):12-21.

Green, C. J.; Knight, J.; Precious, S.; and Simpkin, S. 1981. Ketamine alone and combined with diazepam or xylazine in laboratory animals: A 10-year experience. Lab. Anim. 15:163-170.

Habermann, R. T., and Williams, F. P. 1957. The efficacy of some piperazine compounds and stylomycin in drinking water for the removal of oxyurids from mice and rats and a method of critical testing of anthelmintics. Proc. Anim. Care Panel 7(2):89-97.

Hafez, E. S. E. 1970. Rabbits. In Reproduction and Breeding Techniques for Laboratory Animals, E. S. E. Hafez, ed., 273-298. Lea and Febiger, Philadelphia.

Hagen, K. W. 1974. Colony husbandry. In The Biology of The Laboratory Rabbit, S. H. Weisbroth, R. E. Flatt, and A. L. Kraus, eds., 23-47. Academic Press, New York.

Hagen, K. W., and Gorham, J. R. 1972. Dermatomycoses in fur animals: Chinchilla, ferret, mink, and rabbit. VM/SAC 67:43-48.

Hall, R. N. 1973. Biohazards associated with simian viruses. In Biohazards in Biomedical Research, A. Hellman, M. N. Oxman, and R. Pollack, eds., 3-40. Cold Springs Harbor Laboratory, Cold Springs Harbor, New York.

Hammond, J., Jr., and Chesterman, F. C. 1976. The ferret. In The UFAW Handbook on the Care and Management of Laboratory Animals, 5th ed., ed. UFAW, Churchill Livingstone, Edinburgh.

Harkness, J. E. 1982. Practical primatology: The ASLAP continuing education conference in Bastrop. Synapse 14(3):23-27.

Harkness, J. E., and Ferguson, F. G. 1982. Bacterial, mycoplasmal, and mycotic diseases of the lymphoreticular, musculoskeletal, cardiovascular, and endocrine systems. In The Mouse in Biomedical Research, vol. 2, H. L. Foster, J. D. Small, and J. G. Fox, eds., 83-97. Academic Press, New York.

Harkness J. E., and Wagner, J. E. 1977. The Biology and Medicine of Rabbits and Rodents. Lea and Febiger, Philadelphia.

______. 1983. The Biology and Medicine of Rabbits and Rodents, 2nd ed. Lea and Febiger, Philadelphia.

Held, J. R. 1981a. Breeding and use of nonhuman primates in the USA. Int. J. Stud. Anim. Probl. 2(1):27-37.

______. 1981b. Summary: Ectromelia (mousepox) in the United States. Lab. Anim. Sci. 31:630-632.

Hinsch, H., and Gandal, C. P. 1969. The effects of etorphine (M-99), oxymorphone hydrochloride, and meperidine hydrochloride in reptiles. Copeia 2:404-405.

Hoag, W. G. 1961. Oxyuriasis in laboratory mouse colonies. Am. J. Vet. Res. 22:150-153.

Hoffman, R. A. 1968. Hibernation and effects of low temperature. In The Golden Hamster: Its Biology and Use in Medical Research, R. A. Hoffman, P. F. Robinson, and H. Magalhaes, 25-39. Iowa State University Press, Ames.

Holmes, D. D.; Kosanke, S. D.; and White, G. L. 1980. Fatal enterobiasis in a chimpanzee. J. Am. Vet. Med. Assoc. 177:911-913.

Hsu, C. K. 1979. Parasitic diseases, In The Laboratory Rat, vol. 1, H. J. Baker, J. R. Lindsey, and S. H. Weisbroth, eds., 307-331. Academic Press, New York.

Hughes, H. C. 1981. Anesthesia of laboratory animals. Lab Anim. 10(5):40-56.

Hull, S. W. 1977. The ferret. Lab Anim. 6(6):57-58.

Hunt, R. D., and Melendez, L. U. 1969. Herpesvirus infections of nonhuman primates. Lab. Anim. Care 19:221-234.

Jacobson, E. R. 1981. Diseases of reptiles, part II: Infectious diseases. Compend. Contin. Educ. 3:195-199.

Jacoby, R. O.; Bhatt, N.; and Jonas, A. M. 1979. Viral diseases. In The Laboratory Rat, vol 1, H. J. Baker, J. R. Lindsey, and S. H. Weisbroth eds., 272-306. Academic Press, New York.

Jaslow, B. W.; Ringler, D. H.; Rush, H. G.; and Glorioso, J. C. 1981. Pasteurella associated rhinitis of rabbits: Efficacy of penicillin therapy. Lab. Anim. Sci. 31:382-385.

Johnson, D. K.; Russell, R. J.; Stunkard, J. A. 1981. A Guide to Diagnosis, Treatment, and Husbandry of Nonhuman Primates. Veterinary Medicine Publ., Edwardsville, Kans.

Kaplan, H. M. 1963. Effects of ether and of sodium pentobarbital upon turtle blood. Lab. Anim. Care 13:181-185.

Karlstrom, E. L., and Cook, S. F. 1955. Notes on snake anesthesia. Copeia 1:57-58.

Keeler, R. F., and Young, S. 1979. Role of vitamin E in the etiology of spontaneous hemorrhagic necrosis of the central nervous system of fetal hamsters. Teratology 20:127-132.

Kociba, G. J., and Caputo, C. A. 1981. Aplastic anemia associated with estrus in pet ferrets. J. Am. Vet. Med. Assoc. 178:1293-1294.

Koehn, C. J. 1966. The feeding of baboons, Papio cynocephalus and P. doguera. Lab. Anim. Care 16:178-184.

Kohn, D. F., and MacKenzie, W. F. 1980. Inner ear disease characterized by rolling in C3H mice. J. Am. Vet. Med. Assoc. 177:815-817.

Kraft, L. M. 1982. Viral diseases of the digestive system. In The Mouse in Biomedical Research, vol. 2, H. L. Foster, J. D. Small, and J. G. Fox, eds., 159-191, Academic Press, New York.

Krushak, D. H. 1970. Application of preventive health measures to curtail chimpanzee-associated infectious hepatitis in handlers. Lab. Anim. Care 20:52-56.

Kuhn, U. S. G., and Arko, R. J. 1974. Repeated ketamine anesthesia in the chimpanzee. J. Am. Vet. Med. Assoc. 165:838-839.

Kupper, J. L.; Casey, H. W.; and Johnson, D. K. 1970. Experimental yaba and benign epidermal monkeypox in rhesus monkeys. Lab. Anim. Care 20:979-988.

La Regina, M.; Fales, W. H.; and Wagner, J. E. 1980. Effects of antibiotic treatment on the occurrence of experimentally induced proliferative ileitis of hamsters. Lab. Anim. Sci. 30:38-41.

Lee, K. J.; Lang, C. M.; Hughes, H. C.; and Hartshorn, R. D. 1981. Psorergatic mange (acari: Psorergatidae) of the stumptail macaque (Macaca artoides). Lab. Anim. Sci. 31:77-79.

Lennette, E. H. 1973. Potential hazards posed by nonviral agents. In Biohazards in Biological Research, A. Hellman, M. N. Oxman, and R. Pollack, eds., 47-62. Cold Spring Harbor Laboratory, Cold Spring Harbor, New York.

Lentsch, R. H.; McLaughlin, R. M.; Wagner, J. E.; and Day, T. J. 1982. Campylobacter fetus subspecies jejuni isolated from Syrian hamsters with proliferative ileitis. Lab. Anim. Sci. 32:511-514.

Lewis, C., and Gray, J. E. 1961. Experimental Leptospira pomona infection in the Mongolian gerbil (Meriones unguiculatus). J. Infect. Dis. 109:194-204.

Lindsey, J. R., and Fox, R. R. 1974. Inherited diseases and variations. In The Biology of the Laboratory Rabbit, S. H. Weisbroth, R. E. Flatt, and A. L. Kraus, eds., 377-401. Academic Press, New York.

Lindsey, J. R., and Melby, E. C., Jr. 1966. Naturally occurring primary cutaneous tuberculosis in the rhesus monkey. Lab. Anim. Care 16:369-385.

Lindsey, J. R., Cassell, G. H., and Davidson, M. K. 1982. Mycoplasmal and other bacterial diseases of the respiratory system. In The Mouse in Biomedical Research, vol. 2, H. L. Foster, J. D. Small, and J. G. Fox, eds., 21-41. Academic Press, New York.

Lumb, W. B., and Jones, E. W. 1973. Veterinary Anesthesia, Lea and Febiger, 179-244. Philadelphia, Pa.

McBride, D. F.; Stark, D. M.; and Walberg, J. A. 1981. An outbreak of staphylococcal furunculosis in nude mice. Lab. Anim. Sci. 31:270-272.

McClure, H. M.; Chapman, W. L., Jr.; Hooper, B. E.; Smith, F. G.; and Fletcher, O. J. 1978. The digestive system. In Pathology of Laboratory Animals, vol. 1, K. Benirschke, F. M. Garner, and T. C. Jones, eds., 176-317. Springer-Verlag, New York.

McDonald, S. E., and Lavoipierre, M. J. 1980. Trixacarus caviae infestation in two guinea pigs. Lab. Anim. Sci. 30:67-70.

McDougall, P. T.; Wolf, N. S.; Stenback, W. A.; and Trentin, J. J. 1967. Control of Pseudomonas aeruginosa in an experimental mouse colony. Lab. Anim. Care. 17:204-214.

Machlin, L. J.; Garcia, F.; Kuenzig, W.; and Brin, M. 1979. Antiscorbutic activity of ascorbic acid phosphate in the rhesus monkey and the guinea pig. Am. J. Clin. Nutr. 32:325-331.

McPherson, C. W. 1973. Biology and use in research. In The Mouse, ACLAM Laboratory Animal Medicine and Science Series coord., G. L. Van Hoosier, Jr., 1-20. University of Washington, Seattle.

Magalhaes, H. 1968. Gross anatomy. In The Golden Hamster: Its Biology and Use in Medical Research, R. A. Hoffman, P. F. Robinson, and H. Magalhaes, eds., 91-109. Iowa State University Press, Ames.

Marcus, L. C. 1977. Parasitic diseases of captive reptiles. In Current Veterinary Therapy VI: Small Animal Practice, R. W. Kirk, ed., 801-806. Saunders, Philadelphia.

______. 1980. Bacterial infections in reptiles. In Reproductive Biology and Diseases of Captive Reptiles, J. B. Murphy and J. T. Collins, eds., 211-221. Meseraull Printing, Lawrence, Kans.

______. 1981. Veterinary Biology and Medicine of Captive Amphibians and Reptiles. Lea and Febiger, Philadelphia.

Marston, J. H. 1976. The Mongolian gerbil. In The UFAW Handbook on the Care and Management of Laboratory Animals, 5th ed., ed. UFAW, 236-274. Churchill, Livingstone, Edinburgh.

Marston, J. H., and Chang, M. C. 1965. The breeding, management, and reproductive physiology of the Mongolian gerbil (Meriones unguiculatus). Lab. Anim. Care, 15:34-48.

Martin, D. P.; Darrow, C. C.; Valerio, D. A.; and Leiseca, S. A. 1972. Methods of anesthesia in nonhuman primates. Lab. Anim. Sci. 22:837-843.

Meckley, P. E., and Zwicker, G. M. 1979. Naturally occurring neoplasms in the Mongolian gerbil, Meriones unguiculatus. Lab. Anim. 13:203-206.

Melby, E. C., and Altman, N. H., eds. 1976. Handbook of Laboratory Animal Science, vol. 3. CRC Press, Cleveland.

Merck Veterinary Manual, 5th ed. 1979. Merck, Rahway, N.J.

Mia, A. S.; Kravcak, D. M.; and Cassell, G. H. 1981. Detection of Mycoplasma pulmonis antibody in rats and mice by a rapid micro enzyme-linked immunosorbent assay. Lab. Anim. Sci. 31:356-359.

Miller, W. R., and Merton, D. A. 1982. Dirofilariasis in a ferret. J. Am. Vet. Med. Assoc. 180:1103-1104.

Moskow, B. S.; Wasserman, B. H.; and Rennert, M. C. 1968. Spontaneous periodontal disease in the Mongolian gerbil. J. Periodontal. Res. 3:59-83.

Mulder, J. B.; Whitney, R. A., Jr.; and McPherson, C. W. 1977. Biology and use. In Nonhuman Primates, ACLAM Laboratory Animal Medicine and Science Series, coord., G. L. Van Hoosier, Jr., 17-38. University of Washington, Seattle.

Mulder, J. B.; Johnson, H. B.; McKee, G. S.; Sellers, S. E. 1979. Anesthesia with Ketaset Plus in guinea pigs and hamsters. VM/SAC 74:1807-1808.

Murphy, J. B. 1973. The use of macrolide antibiotic tylosin in the treatment of reptilian respiratory infections. Br. J. Herpetolog. 4:317-321.

Napier, J. R., and Napier, P. H. 1967. A Handbook of Living Primates. Academic Press, New York.

National Cancer Institute. 1979. Biological Hazards in the Nonhuman Primate Laboratory. Enviro Control, Rockville, Md.

Navia, J. M., and Hunt, C. E. 1976. Nutrition, nutritional diseases, and nutrition research application. In The Biology of the Guinea Pig, J. E. Wagner and P. J. Manning, eds., 235-267. Academic Press, New York.

Nguyen, H. T.; Moreland, A. F.; and Shields, R. P. 1979. Urolithiasis in ferrets (Mustela putorius). Lab. Anim. Sci. 29:243-245.

Norris, M. L., and Adams, C. E. 1972. Incidence of cystic ovaries and reproductive performance in the Mongolian gerbil, Meriones unguiculatus. Lab. Anim. 6:337-342.

Ohshima, K.; Shen, D. T.; Henson, J. B.; and Gorham, J. R. 1978. Comparison of the lesions of Aleutian disease in mink and hypergammaglobulinemia in ferrets. Am. J. Vet. Res. 39:653-657.

Orcutt, R. P. 1980. Bacterial diseases: Agents, pathology, diagnosis, and effects on research. Lab Anim. 9(3):28-42.

Parker, J. C., and Richter, C. B. 1982. Viral diseases of the respiratory system. In The Mouse in Biomedical Research, vol. 2, H. L. Foster, J. D. Small, and J. G. Fox, eds., 110-158. Academic Press, New York.

Pasteurella-resistant rabbits. 1981. J. Appl. Rabbit Res. 4(3):56.

Patton, N. M. 1979. What every practitioner should know about rabbits and rodents. Calif. Vet. 33(5):25-33.

______. 1981. Isolation of an adenovirus from rabbits with diarrhea. J. Appl. Rabbit Res. 4(1):21.

Patton, N. M., and Cheeke, P. R. 1981. A precautioniary note on high fiber levels and mucoid enteritis. J. Appl. Rabbit Res. 4(3):56.

Patton, N. M.; Holmes, H. T.; Riggs, R. J.; and Cheeke, P. R. 1978. Enterotoxemia in rabbits. Lab. Anim. Sci. 28:536-540.

Peardon, D. L.; Tufts, J. M.; and Eschenroeder, H. C. 1966. Experimental treatment of laboratory rats naturally infected with Trichosomoides crassicauda. Invest. Urol. 4:215-219.

Peckham, J. C.; Cole, J. R.; Chapman, W. L., Jr.; Malone, J. B., Jr.; McCall, J. W.; and Thompson, P. E. 1974. Staphylococcal dermatitis in Mongolian gerbils (Meriones unguiculatus). Lab. Anim. Sci. 24:43-47.

Peters, L. J. 1981. The guinea pig: An overview, part II. Compend. Contin. Educ. 3(5):403-410.

Pond, D. L.; Newcomer, C. E.; and Anver, M. R. 1982. Acute gastric dilatation in nonhuman primates: Review and case studies. Vet. Pathol. 19:126-133.

Port, C. D.; Richter, W. R.; and Moise, S. M. 1970. Tyzzer's disease in the gerbil (Meriones unguiculatus). Lab. Anim. Care 20:109-111.

Post, K., and Saunders, J. R. Topical treatment of experimental ringworm in guinea pigs with griseofulvin in dimethylsulfoxide. Can. Vet. J., 20:45-48.

Potkay, S.; Ganaway, J. R.; Rogers, N. G.; and Kinard, R. 1966. An epizootic of measles in a colony of rhesus monkeys (Macaca mulatta). Am. J. Vet. Res. 27:331-334.

Randall, L. O., and Selitto, J. J. 1957. A method for measurement of analgesic activity on inflamed tissue. Arch. Int. Pharmacodyn. Ther. 111:409-419.

Raphael, B. L. 1981. Pet rabbit medicine. Compend. Contin. Educ. 3(1):60-64.

Rehg, J. E., and Lu, Y. S. 1981. Clostridium difficile colitis in a rabbit following antibiotic therapy for pasteurellosis. J. Am. Vet. Med. Assoc. 179:1296-1297.

Rehg, J. E., and Pakes, S. P. 1981. Clostridium difficile antitoxin neutralization of cecal toxin(s) from guinea pigs with penicillin-associated colitis. Lab. Anim. Sci. 31:156-159.

Rich, S. T. 1968. The Mongolian gerbil (Meriones unguiculatus) in research. Lab. Anim. Care 18:235-243.

Robbins, S. L. 1974. Pathogenic Basis of Disease. Saunders, Philadelphia.

Rosenberg, D. P.; Lerche, N. W.; and Henrickson, R. V. 1980. Yersinia pseudotuberculosis infection in a group of Macaca fascicularis. J. Am. Vet. Med. Assoc. 177:818-819.

Ross, C. R.; Wagner, J. E.; Wightman, S. R.; and Dill, S. E. 1980. Experimental transmission of Syphacia muris among rats, mice, hamsters, and gerbils. Lab. Anim. Sci. 30:35-37.

Rossoff, I. F. 1974. Handbook of Veterinary Drugs. Springer-Verlag, New York.

Ruch, T. C. 1959. Disease of Laboratory Primates. W. B. Saunders, Philadelphia.

Rush, H. G. 1982. Personal communication.

Russell, R. J.; Johnson, D. K.; and Stunkard, J. A. 1981. A Guide to Diagnosis, Treatment, and Husbandry of Pet Rabbits and Rodents. Veterinary Medicine Publ., Edwardsville, Kans.

Ryland, L. M. 1982. Remission of estrus-associated anemia following ovariohysterectomy and multiple blood transfusions in a ferret. J. Am. Vet. Med. Assoc. 181:820-822.

Ryland, L. M., and Bernard, S. L. 1983. A clinical guide to the pet ferret. Compend. Contin. Educ. 5:25-32.

Ryland, L. M., and Gorham, J. R. 1978. The ferret and its diseases. J. Am. Vet. Med. Assoc. 173:1154-1158.

Schuchman, S. M. 1977. Individual care and treatment of rabbits, mice, rats, guinea pigs, hamsters and gerbils. In Current Veterinary Therapy VI: Small Animal Practice, R. W. Kirk, ed., 726-756. Saunders, Philadelphia.

Schwarzbrott, S. S.; Wagner, J. E.; and Frisk, C. S. 1974. Demodicosis in the Mongolian gerbil (Meriones unguiculatus): A case report. Lab. Anim. Sci. 24:666-668.

Schwentker, V. 1963. The gerbil, a new laboratory animal. Ill. Vet. 6:5-9.

Sebesteny, A. 1979. Syrian hamsters. In Handbook of Diseases of Laboratory Animals: Diagnosis and Treatment, J. M. Hime, and P. N. O'Donoghue, eds., 111-136. Heinemann Veterinary Books, London.

Sedgwick, C. J. 1982. Spaying the rabbit. Mod. Vet. Pract. 63:401-403.

Sedgwick, C. J.; Robinson, P. T.; and Lochner, F. K. 1975. Zoonoses: A zoo's concern. J. Am. Vet. Med. Assoc. 167:828-829.

Seibold, H. R.; Perrin, E. A., Jr.; and Garner, A. C. 1970. Pneumonia associated with Bordetella bronchiseptica in Callicebus species primates. Lab. Anim. Care 20:456-461.

Setser, M. D. 1983. Personal communication.

Shadduck, J. A., and Pakes, S. P. 1978. Protozoal and metazoal diseases. In Pathology of Laboratory Animals, vol. 2, K. Benirshke, F. M. Garner, and T. C. Jones eds., 1588-1696, Springer-Verlag, New York.

Sheffield, F. W., and Beveridge, E. 1962. Prophylaxis of "wet tail" in hamsters. Nature 196:294-295.

Simmons, M. L., and Brick, J. O. 1970. The Laboratory Mouse: Selection and Management. Prentice-Hall, Englewood Cliffs, N. J.

Simmons, M. L.; Williams, H. E.; and Wright, E. B. 1965. Therapeutic value of the organic phosphate trichlorfon against Syphacia obvelata in inbred mice. Lab. Anim. Care 15:382-385.

Sisk, D. B. 1976. Physiology. In The Biology of the Guinea Pig, J. E. Wagner, and P. J. Manning, eds., 63-98. Academic Press, N.Y.

Skulski, G., and Symmers, W. St. C. 1954. Actinomycosis and torulosis in the ferret. J. Comp. Pathol. 64:306-311.

Small, J. D.; Aurelian, L; Squire, R. A.; Strandberg, J. D.; Melby, E. C., Jr.; Turner, T. B.; and Newman, B. 1979. Rabbit cardiomyopathy associated with a virus antigenically related to human coronavirus strain 229E. Am. J. Pathol. 95:709-728.

Smith, S. M., and Kaplan, H. M. 1974. Ketamine-methoxyflurane anesthesia for the mongolian gerbil, *Meriones unguiculatus*. Lab. Anim. 8:213-216.

Sprouse, R. F. 1976. Mycoses. In *The Biology of the Guinea Pig*, J. E. Wagner, and P. J. Manning, eds., 153-161. Academic Press, New York.

Stein, S. 1981. Practical tip. Synapse 14(2):8.

Stookey, J. L., and Moe, J. B. 1978. The respiratory system. In *Pathology of Laboratory Animals*, vol. 1, K. Benirshke, F. M. Garner, and T. C. Jones, eds., 71-113. Springer-Verlag, New York.

Straube, E. F., and Walden, N. B. 1981. Zinc poisoning in ferrets (Mustella *putorius furo*). Lab. Anim. 15:45-47.

Straube, E. F.; Schuster, N. H.; and Sinclair, A. J. 1980. Zinc toxicity in the ferret. J. Comp. Pathol. 90:355-361.

Symmers, W. St. C., and Thomson, A. P. D. 1953. Observations on tuberculosis in the ferret (*Mustela furo* L). J. Comp. Pathol. 63:20-30.

Thornton, P. C.; Wright, P. A.; Sacra, P. J.; and Goodier, T. E. W. 1979. The ferret, *Mustela putorius furo*, as a new species in toxicology. Lab. Anim. 13:119-124.

Timm, K. I.; Thomas, N. J., and Frye, F. L. 1979. Adenocarcinoma in a young rabbit (an atypical case). VM/SAC 74:1003-1007.

Unay, E. S., and Davis, B. J. 1980. Treatment of *Syphacia obvelata* in the Syrian hamster (*Mesocricetus auratus*) with piperazine citrate. Am. J. Vet. Res. 41:1899-1900.

USDA. 1976. *Domestic Rabbits: Diseases and Parasites*, Agriculture Handbook 490. Washington, D. C.

Utroska, B., and Austin, W. L. 1979. Bilateral cataracts in a ferret. VM/SAC 74:1176-1177.

Van Hoosier, G. L., Jr., and Robinette, L. R. 1976. Viral and chlamydial diseases. In *The Biology of the Guinea Pig*, J. E. Wagner and P. J. Manning, eds., 137-152. Academic Press, New York.

Van Riper, D. C.; Day, P. W.; Fineg, J.; and Prine, J. R. 1966. Intestinal parasites of recently imported chimpanzees. Lab. Anim. Care 16:360-363.

Vetterling, J. M. 1976. Protozoan parasites. In *The Biology of the Guinea Pig*, J. E. Wagner and P. J. Manning, eds., 163-196. Academic Press, New York.

Vincent, A. L., and Ash, L. R. 1978. Further observations on spontaneous neoplasms in the Mongolian gerbil *Meriones unguiculatus*. Lab. Anim. Sci. 28:297-300.

Vincent, A. L., Rodrick, G. E.; and Sodeman, W. A., Jr. 1979. The pathology of the Mongolian gerbil (*Meriones unguiculatus*): A review. Lab. Anim. Sci. 29:645-651.

Vondruska, J. F. 1965. Phencyclidine anesthesia in baboons. J. Am. Vet. Med. Assoc. 147:1073-1074.

Wagner, J. E. 1970. Control of mouse pinworms, *Syphacia obvelata*, utilizing dichlorvos. Lab. Anim. Care 20:39-44.

_______. 1976. Miscellaneous disease conditions of guinea pigs. In *The Biology of the Guinea Pig*, J. E. Wagner and P. J. Manning, 227-234. Academic Press, New York.

_______. 1979. Guinea pigs. In *Handbook of Diseases of Laboratory Animals: Diagnosis and Treatment*, J. M. Hime and P. N. O'Donoghue, eds., 137-162. Heinemann Veterinary Books, London.

Wagner, J. E., and Daynes, R. A. 1981. Observations of an outbreak of mousepox in laboratory mice in 1979 at the University of Utah Medical Center. Lab. Anim. Sci. 31:565-569.

Wallach, J. D. 1969. Medical care of reptiles. J. Am. Vet. Med. Assoc. 155:1017-1034.

Wallach, J. D. and Hoessle, C. 1970. M-99 as an immobilizing agent in poikilotherms. VM/SAC 65:163-167.

Walshaw, O. W. 1983. Reptilian management and medical care. Anim. Health Tech. 4:147-154.

Wass, J. A.; Keene, J. R.; and Kaplan, H. M. 1974. Ketamine-methoxyflurane anesthesia for rabbits. Am. J. Vet. Res. 35:317-318.

Wechsler, S. J. 1983. Blood collection techniques and normal values for ferrets, rabbits, and rodents. VM/SAC 78:713-717.

Weisbroth, S. H. 1974. Neoplastic diseases. In The Biology of the Laboratory Rabbit, S. H. Weisbroth, R. E. Flatt, and A. L. Kraus, eds., 332-375. Academic Press, New York.

______. 1979. Bacterial and mycotic diseases. In The Laboratory Rat, vol. 1, H. J. Baker, J. R. Lindsey, and S. H. Weisbroth, eds., 193-241. Academic Press, New York.

Weisbroth, S. H., and Fudens, J. H. 1972. Use of ketamine hydrochloride as an anesthetic in laboratory rabbits, rats, mice, and guinea pigs. Lab. Anim. Sci. 22:904-906.

Weisbroth, S. H., and Scher, S. 1971. Trichosomoides crassicauda infection of a commercial rat breeding colony. II. Drug screening for anthelmintic activity and field trials with methyridine. Lab. Anim. Sci. 21:213-219.

Welch, P. L. 1983. Personal communication.

Wescott, R. B. 1976. Helminth parasites. In The Biology of the Guinea Pig, J. E. Wagner and P. J. Manning, eds., 197-200. Academic Press, New York.

White, G. L., and Cummings, J. F. 1979. A comparison of ketamine and ketamine-xylazine in the baboon. VM/SAC 74:392-396.

White, G. L., and Holmes, D. D. 1976. A comparison of ketamine and the combination ketamine-xylazine for effective surgical anesthesia in the rabbit. Lab. Anim. Sci. 26:804-806.

Whitney, R. A., Jr. 1975. Important primate diseases (biohazards and zoonoses). In Cancer Research Safety Monographs 2:23-52.

______. 1979. Primate medicine and husbandry. Small Anim. Pract. 9:429-445.

Whitney, R. A., Jr., and Kruckenberg, S. M. 1967. Pentastomid infection associated with peritonitis in mangabey monkeys. J. Am. Vet. Med. Assoc. 151:907-908.

Whitney, R. A., Jr., and Mulder, J. B. 1977. Introduction and taxonomy. In Nonhuman Primates. ACLAM Laboratory Animal Medicine and Science Series, coord. G. L. Van Hoosier, Jr., 1-16. University of Washington, Seattle.

Whitney, R. A., Jr.; Johnson, D. J.; and Cole, W. C. 1973. Laboratory Primate Handbook. Academic Press, New York.

Whitney, R. A., Jr.; Mulder, J. B.; and Johnson, D. K. 1977. Nonhuman primates: Bacterial diseases. In Nonhuman Primates. ACLAM Laboratory Animal Medicine and Science Series, coord. G. L. Van Hoosier, Jr., 77-94. University of Washington, Seattle.

Wightman, S. R.; Wagner, J. E.; and Corwin, R. M. 1978. Syphacia obvelata in the Mongolian gerbil (Meriones unguiculatus): Natural occurrence and experimental transmission. Lab. Anim. Sci. 28:51-54.

Wightman, S. R.; Mann, P. C.; and Wagner, J. E. 1980. Dihydrostreptomycin toxicity in the Mongolian gerbil, *Meriones unguiculatus*. *Lab. Anim. Sci.* 30:71-75.

Williams, C. S. F. 1976. *Practical Guide to Laboratory Animals*. C. V. Mosby, St. Louis, Mo.

_______. 1979. Guinea pigs and rabbits. *Small Anim. Pract.* 9(3):487-497.

Willis, L. S., and Barrow, M. V. 1971. The ferret (*Mustela putorius furo* L) as a laboratory animal. *Lab. Anim. Sci.* 21:712-716.

Willis, R. A., Jensen, M. 1979. A preliminary report on cause and prevention of mucoid enteritis. *Domest. Rabbits* 7:20-22.

Wills, J. H. 1968. Pharmacology. In *The Golden Hamster: Its Biology and Use in Medical Research*, R. A. Hoffman, P. F. Robinson, and H. Magalhaes, eds., 203-208. Iowa State University Press, Ames.

Woolfson, M. W.; Foran, J. A.; Freedman, H. M.; Moore, P. A.; Shulman, L. B.; and Schnitman, P. A. 1980. Immobilization of baboons (*Papio anubis*) using ketamine and diazepam. *Lab. Anim. Sci.* 30:902-904.

Young, R., and Kaplan, H. M. 1960. Anesthesia of turtles with chlorpromazine and sodium pentobarbital. *Proc. Anim. Care Panel* 10(2):57-62.

Zajac, A.; Williams, J. F.; and Williams, C. S. F. 1980. Mange caused by *Trixacarus caviae* in guinea pigs. *J. Am. Vet. Med. Assoc.* 177:900-903.

Zwicker, G. M., and Carlton, W. W. 1974. Spontaneous squamous cell carcinoma in a ferret. *J. Wildl. Dis.* 10:213-216.

INDEX